"Alisa Vitti is my go-to hormone expert and yes, us younger women need one! She has helped me with my cycle, my skin, and my energy—all with food!"

—Gabrielle Bernstein, *New York Times* bestselling author of *May Cause Miracles*

"Alisa is a management guru for the female body. She makes hormonal health approachable and fun!"

—Kris Carr, *New York Times* bestselling author of *Crazy Sexy Kitchen*

"Alisa Vitti's approachable blend of the science of hormones, with healthy food and lifestyle choices, creates a vibrant, radiant you from the inside out. Alisa's WomanCode method reminds us there is always movement in balance and helps us find the ease in our constantly changing cycle."

—Tara Stiles, founder of Strala Yoga and bestselling author of *Yoga Cures* and *Slim Calm Sexy Yoga*

"WomanCode is a brilliant nutrition program for all of the hormonal challenges that prevent women from looking and feeling their best. Alisa Vitti provides a practical food approach to ease your periods, improve your fertility, and get more energy for your life! Let Alisa guide you to eat right from your brain to your ovaries and start feeling better!"

—JJ Virgin, *New York Times* bestselling author of *The Virgin Diet*

"Alisa is a thought leader when it comes to providing women with the healthcare they really need. Her revolutionary approach will transform your body and your life. More GYNS should prescribe her system to their patients."

—Dr. Frank Lipman, founder of Eleven Eleven Wellness Center and author of *Revive*

"Alisa provides women key information about their bodies and hormones and *WomanCode* is a must-read for all women who want to optimize their fertility and hormonal well-being."

—Christy Jones, founder of ExtendFertility.com

"Alisa Vitti's must-read book gives you back your woman-power. *WomanCode* will put you in control of your reproductive health in a natural way. Your ovaries will thank you for it."

—Gloria Feldt, author of *No Excuses: 9 Ways Women Can Change How We Think About Power* and former national director of Planned Parenthood

"Alisa Vitti teaches you to unlock the 'Woman Code,' also known as your endocrine system, so you can control your hormones naturally, rather than letting them control you. Armed with knowledge about how to balance your hormones with diet and lifestyle changes, you'll be able to take your health into your own hands and relish being a woman instead of cursing your gender. A must-read!"

—Dr. Lissa Rankin, OB/GYN and author of *Mind Over Medicine: Scientific Proof You Can Heal Yourself*

"*WomanCode* is an extraordinary food-based prescription for your period, fertility, and lackluster sex drive. In her authoritative book, Alisa Vitti shares her rigorous functional nutrition protocol so you can nourish your ovaries and optimize your hormones naturally. Vitti is breaking new ground by replacing our broken system of women's health with her novel approach."

—Dr. Sara Gottfried, OB/GYN, and author of *The Hormone Cure*

"I am an expert in helping my A-List celebrity clients create the body they want. I see how much hormonal fluctuations affect a woman's workout, mood, energy, and ability to achieve her goals. Women must learn how their insides determine their outsides and there is a way to eat for hormonal health and more beautiful bodies."

—Ary Nunez, Nike athlete, NFL trainer, and founder of ArysAmerica.com

"*WomanCode* is your ultimate hormonal handbook. Alisa Vitti is truly a women's health visionary for the next generation. She inspires women to take control of their bodies and experience much greater health and happiness than ever before!"

—Joshua Rosenthal, founder and director of the Institute for Integrative Nutrition

"*WomanCode* is a revolutionary, step-by-step guide that will help countless women balance their hormones, love their bodies, and feel great in their own skin. For too long, women have feared and battled their bodies, not understanding how to work in concert with their hormones. Alisa Vitti's tested, brilliant strategies are the cure you've been looking for to end your battle with your body. *WomanCode* gives you the tools to create the necessary shift so you can own your body, reclaim your reproductive health, and take responsibility for your well-being."

—Alexandra Jamieson, author of *The Great American Detox Diet*

"Finally! It's here!! Alisa has researched and created a comprehensive guided tour down the yellow brick road of woman's sparkling health and well-being. Science meets woman! At last!!"

—Regena Thomashauer, author of *Mama Gena's School of Womanly Arts*

"*WomanCode* will empower you to get your hormones in proper balance and put your body in an optimally fertile state. Alisa Vitti's whole food-based protocol will help you nourish your womb and bloom into pregnancy."

—Latham Thomas, bestselling author of *Mama Glow: A Hip Guide to Your Fabulous Abundant Pregnancy*

"With all the empowered choices modern women have today, how, when, and if we become mothers—if that's what we want—is often out of our control. Whether at late-age fertility and still looking for love and the right partner, suffering from biological infertility, or simply not prepared to consider motherhood today, read this book *now*. *WomanCode* is the right choice for women who want to power-up their female health and preserve and strengthen their fertility, now and for the future."

—Melanie Notkin, founder of Savvy Auntie, bestselling author of *Savvy Auntie,* and upcoming author of *Otherhood* (early 2014)

"Alisa has a deep understanding, wisdom, and true knowledge for the female body . . . she loves it with all her soul and her love has led her to do her extensive research, which now gives us all a guide to serve our unique biology and rhythm. This book is a breakthrough to your hormonal health. Read it, carry in your purse, keep it by your bathtub, devour its wisdom. Your body will love you for it."

—Agapi Stassinopoulos, author of *Unbinding the Heart*

"Alisa Vitti does a body good. She's a wizard when it comes to women's inner and outer workings. Her groundbreaking approach to hormonal cycles contains secrets I only wish I'd known when I was growing up. And she teaches them in a fun, fascinating way—a must-read for anyone with ovaries . . . and without!"

—Ophira Edut, author of *Love Zodiac* and *Body Outlaws*

"Women want the best when it comes to feeding their children, but what we must learn is how to feed our bodies to be the best moms we can be. Hormonal imbalances zap your energy, your moods, your ability to enjoy your children in addition to all of the real health concerns they bring. *WomanCode* will teach you how to eat for your hormones and create a better future for your family. Every woman should be a part of Alisa Vitti's vision for women's health."

—Shazi Visram, founder and CEO of Happy Family Foods

"As a husband and father, I want to see the women in my life happy and thriving. *WomanCode* is the definitive guide for women's hormonal health. If you want to have a more successful relationship with the women in your life, get this book for yourself and the women you love."

—Eric Handler, founder of PositivelyPositive.com

"In *WomanCode*, Alisa has found a way to demystify both the magic and the science of hormones. I feel blessed to call Alisa friend and in this book, jam-packed with easy and tangible tools for befriending your body, I feel like we are just having one of our fabulous female powwows, and as always with Alisa, I leave feeling empowered and awesome in my body!"

—Alysia Reiner, actress, filmmaker, mother, alysiareiner.com

"Alisa Vitti is a triumvirate of one part science, one part sexy, and one part pure empowered female. She writes from a place of knowledge *and* wisdom—both a hard-won education and an invaluable personal experience of miraculous transformation. *WomanCode* is your body's bible. The body speaks a language that we can learn to interpret to heal and become clearer channels for our soul-work in the world. Alisa speaks body. She relates with ease and from the depths of her own transformational experience how understanding the language of the body effortlessly allows optimal health and healing to flow through us. Fall in love with your body, from your hormones to your adrenal glands, and remember again a truth we are all ready to live: the body is a sacred temple. "

—Meggan Watterson, author of *Reveal*

"*WomanCode* is part wakeup call and part godsend. Alisa Vitti seamlessly meshes science, compassion, story, and solutions in this wise, practical guide to a woman's hormonal health. The protocol outlined in these pages will heal women who've struggled with their hormones for years and healthy women wanting to enhance their lives alike. This book is part of the healthcare revolution that is needed so deeply. Read it and become a part of healing women and healing the planet."

—Kate Northrup, author of *Money: A Love Story*

"Your sex drive needs to be fed properly for it to thrive. While bioidentical hormones may help, *WomanCode* shows you how interconnected your hormonal health truly is and how you can improve your mood and libido from the inside out!"

—Jennifer Landa, M.D., OB/GYN, and author of *The Sex Drive Solution for Women*

"I believe in an integrative approach when it comes to gynecology. *WomanCode* addresses the underlying causes to your most challenging reproductive and hormonal symptoms and gives you jewels that work to restore you. In her elegant and effective food-based functional nutrition protocol, Alisa Vitti shows you how you can have your hormones working for you, not against you!"

—Dr. Anna Cabeca, DO, OB/GYN, FACOG

"Buy this book and follow its suggestions and I can promise you that *WomanCode* will do more for your love life than an aphrodisiac, will bring you more joy than a hot fudge sundae, and will help you have all the energy you need to do everything you dream of. For real! Not only that, it's simple, safe, delicious, and easy. What are you waiting for? Jump in and join the women who are nourishing themselves and their WomanCode."

—Susun S. Weed, herbalist and author, *New Menopausal Years the Wise Woman Way* and *Down There: Sexual and Reproductive Health the Wise Woman Way*

WomanCode

WOMAN CODE

PERFECT YOUR CYCLE, AMPLIFY
YOUR FERTILITY, SUPERCHARGE
YOUR SEX DRIVE, AND BECOME
A POWER SOURCE

Alisa Vitti, HHC, AADP

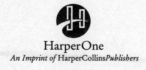

HarperOne
An Imprint of HarperCollinsPublishers

HarperOne

WOMANCODE: *Perfect Your Cycle, Amplify Your Fertility, Supercharge Your Sex Drive, and Become a Power Source.* Copyright © 2013 by Alisa Vitti. All rights reserved. Printed in the United States of America. No part of this book may be used or reproduced in any manner whatsoever without written permission except in the case of brief quotations embodied in critical articles and reviews. For information address HarperCollins Publishers, 10 East 53rd Street, New York, NY 10022.

HarperCollins books may be purchased for educational, business, or sales promotional use. For information, please e-mail the Special Markets Department at SPsales@harpercollins.com.

HarperCollins website: http://www.harpercollins.com

HarperCollins®, ▟®, and HarperOne™ are trademarks of HarperCollins Publishers

Designed by Terry McGrath

FIRST EDITION

Library of Congress Cataloging-in-Publication Data
Vitti, Alisa.
WomanCode : perfect your cycle, amplify your fertility, supercharge your sex drive, and become a power source / by Alisa Vitti, HHC, AADP. —First edition.
    pages cm
ISBN 978–0–06–213077–8
1. Menstrual cycle. 2. Fertility, Human. 3. Women—Sexual behavior. I. Title.
II. Title: Woman code.
RG161.V58 2013
618.1—dc23
                2012037240

13 14 15 16 17 RRD(H) 10 9 8 7 6 5 4 3 2

Ex Ovo Omnia

"Everything comes out of an egg."

—WILLIAM HARVEY

This book is dedicated

To my parents for nurturing me in every way and for having
a farm-to-table home long before it was trendy.

To my ovaries for taking me on this amazing journey.

To my nieces, who inspire me to envision
a new future for women's healthcare.

To my readers . . . I lovingly offer this book in service
to your ovaries, your life, and your prosperity.

CONTENTS

Foreword by Christiane Northrup, MD ix
Overview 1

....

Part I UNLOCKING YOUR WOMANCODE

1 *Putting an End to Your Suffering. Period.* 9

2 *When Bad Hormones Happen to Good Women* 31

3 *Girl Meets Body* 53

....

Part II THE WOMANCODE PROTOCOL

4 *Access Your Healing Code* 77

5 *From Vicious Cycle to Delicious Cycle* 141

6 *Life Happens—WomanCode Survival Strategies* 171

....

Part III BECOMING A POWER SOURCE

7 *Optimize Your Fertility* 205

8 *Supercharge Your Sex Drive* 231

9 *Commit to the Feminine Force Within* 257

10 *Staying in the FLO* 283

Appendixes
  Alisa's Medicine Cabinet 291
  WomanCode-Approved Products 295
  Medicinal Foods for Hormonal Symptoms 297

Bibliography 301

Acknowledgments 303

Notes 305

Index 309

FOREWORD

Christiane Northrup, MD, FACOG,
author *Women's Bodies, Women's Wisdom*
and *The Wisdom of Menopause*

Think back to when you were in middle school. Think back to when you got your first period. Was this event something you talked about with your classmates? Your family? And if you had symptoms, such as heavy bleeding, irregular periods, or cramps, was there a wise healer in your life who told you exactly what you needed to do to establish a healthy partnership with your body, your menstrual cycle, and your cyclic lunar wisdom? Did anyone tell you that your periods, the condition of your skin, and the state of your bowel movements were all indicators of how well your hormones were balanced? Did anyone tell you how to find balance naturally?

Were you ever put on birth control pills to "regulate" your periods? Millions of women the world over are subjected to a barrage of medications and synthetic hormonal treatments designed to mask the symptoms of hormonal imbalance that lead to menstrual cycle, fertility, and libido problems in the first place. The most common of these treatments is birth control pills—which result in over fifty different metabolic consequences that further disrupt a woman's hormonal cycle (for example, birth control pills increase the need for folic acid and vitamin B12, two vitamins that are already in short supply in many women).

Giving birth control pills and other medications to women to regulate their periods, improve their fertility, or enhance their sex drive is akin to putting a piece of tape over the flashing indicator light on the dashboard of your car and pretending you have addressed the engine problem rather than looking under the hood and dealing with the underlying issue.

As a board-certified ob/gyn, I spent years and years being indoctrinated into finding better and more sophisticated pieces of tape (in the form of drugs) to put over the indicator lights of women with hormonal imbalances. But I always knew that there had to be a better way. And that is why I wrote *Women's Bodies, Women's Wisdom*, a book that was quite radical at the time of its original publication. Happily for me, many women intuitively knew that drugs and surgery were not the whole answer. Little did I know that I was breaking ground on a trail that Alisa Vitti and others are now making into a superhighway of women's wisdom. In fact, Alisa is part of a new generation of thought-leaders in women's health who are at the forefront of truly assisting women to understand how to best care for and heal their bodies—including having healthy periods, optimal fertility, and a healthy sex drive.

Her protocol is a tried-and-true plan that brings tangible results for women trying to solve their hormonal issues. You'll be excited to read the stories of the women who have used Alisa's approach and have fixed their periods; gotten pregnant successfully; and restored their sex drive, mood, and energy all without drugs or surgery. *WomanCode* is brilliantly organized and scientifically sound—yet free of jargon so that anyone can understand the principles and how to apply them. Alisa's goal is to help you understand your uniquely female biology in a way that will make balancing your hormones second nature to you.

To understand how important Alisa's work on hormonal balance is, beyond her expertise as a holistic health coach, you also need to know something about what I call her "soul qualities." Imagine, if you will, a bright young sixth-grader named Alisa Vitti who was so taken with the hormonal changes in her body she formed a PERIOD club at her school. Yep—a club for her and her middle school pals to bond around their menstrual cycles—one of our Western society's last real taboos. Now THAT takes ovaries. And of course, Alisa's ovaries were quite large and robust—so large and robust, in fact, that she was later diagnosed with what is called PCOS (polycystic ovary syndrome)—a condition characterized by absent periods, stubborn weight gain, unwanted facial hair, and infertility. A condition for which medicine offers very little hope except for birth control pills, blood sugar regulators, ovulation enhancing drugs, and occasional surgery.

But Alisa—being a bright and audacious bulb—decided that she was NOT about to succumb to simply applying "tape" over the flashing indicator lights of her ovaries, and the rest of her endocrine system. Not her. She decided to defy the prognosis that she was given, which was this: PCOS is incurable and you may be infertile and obese the rest of your life. (NOTE: not all women with PCOS have weight problems, but most do.) So instead of going the traditional medical route, as any science geek such as herself would normally have done—Alisa's ovaries led her on a different quest, a quest to find the real cause of her problem. A journey that led her to research intensively the healing properties of foods and how they can be applied to the organs of the endocrine system to bring it all back to balance. She wanted to find real solutions—not just fancier tape for the indicator lights.

And she succeeded brilliantly! She not only reversed her own condition—she has, through her center in NYC and her website, also helped thousands of women around the world end their suffering with period issues, infertility, and low libido. Together they have learned to partner with their bodies, create hormonal harmony, and reclaim their wonderful cyclic wisdom as well as their libido and their fertility. All without expensive drugs and surgery.

You hold in your hands the precious fruit of Alisa's considerable labor to find her own women's wisdom and pass it on to you. You hold in your hands a very clear, practical, user-friendly solution to the most pervasive and all too common gyn problems that legions of women face today. Here are the solutions that your inner wisdom has been seeking all along. You too can follow Alisa's guidance to find your own fertile, comfortable creative flow—in both your body and your life.

I believe that every woman should learn how to be proactive about her hormonal balance by using food as medicine in order for her to flourish in her body and her life. Having watched Alisa and the FLO Living Center grow over the years, I know I am putting you in excellent and experienced hands.

OVERVIEW

There's a silent epidemic happening to women everywhere: hormonal balance is being destroyed. Over twenty million of us suffer from polycystic ovary syndrome (PCOS), fibroids, endometriosis, painful/difficult/heavy periods, and thyroid and adrenal issues. For the first time since their creation, birth control pills are being used to treat girls under the age of seventeen for endocrine-related concerns. In fact, a key message of this book is that not only are young women suffering similar conditions to their mothers and sisters at an earlier age and with much more intensity, but new conditions are arising that women of older generations have not experienced. Hormone replacement therapy is at an all-time high. One in ten couples is infertile, and hysterectomies are still the number-one surgery performed on women.

Modern gynecological care can't keep up with our demands, yet we women are desperate to restore balance, preserve fertility, and maintain youthful hormonal patterns in our bodies.

Hormones affect everything. Have you ever struggled with acne, oily hair, dandruff, dry skin, cramps, headaches, irritability, exhaustion, constipation, irregular cycles, heavy bleeding, clotting, shedding hair, weight gain, anxiety, insomnia, infertility, lowered sex drive, or bizarre food cravings and felt like your body was just irrational? It's not; it's hormonal. Yet women remain mystified at their bodies' seemingly random display of disconnected symptoms, never thinking that they are connected and hormonally based. Mentioning the word "hormones" usually elicits blank stares or comments that it's relevant only to women over fifty. The reality is, hormones influence you in utero, throughout childhood and adolescence, and, most important, right now as you are reading this sentence. Do you know what your hormones are doing, how you might be interfering with their attempts to stay balanced and keep you symptom free, and if you are dealing with an imbalance, where to begin to get your body and your life back? Your health depends on it.

Many of us have the opportunity to have and do it all—but the downside is that while juggling careers, love, travel, and families, we're not giving our bodies the support they need to sustain these demands. Current diet and lifestyle trends afflict women with problems related to their reproductive health. These issues affect us in our teens, conception years, and menopause.

I believe that when women's bodies don't thrive, we fall out of sync with our lives—out of the zone of possibility, and away from our life's purpose. And when we're not healthy and happy, we lose our way. Too many of us are searching for answers to healing and self-empowerment in the wrong places, with the wrong teachers, and suffering needlessly as a result. What we must do is learn how our endocrine systems function, and how to align our feminine selves with our hormones. This will help prevent chronic gynecological issues and guide us toward our fullest lives.

So what's the solution? In this book, I will explain how easy, logical, and enjoyable it is to stop interfering with hormonal balance, which eliminates frustrating symptoms, and then to proactively care for and maintain this balance with my "five-step system" practice. I'll teach you how to restore your body's hormone balance and reset its baseline for years of optimal health and happiness. My protocol, the WomanCode method, works across hormonal conditions in two major ways: 1) it addresses the underlying reasons for hormonal imbalance; and 2) it focuses on using medicinal foods and lifestyle changes to sequentially bring the endocrine system back to optimal functioning. All so you can fix your period, successfully get pregnant, and supercharge your sex drive.

You know how, when everything falls into place, you feel amazing and opportunities drift your way? I've discovered, from both healing myself of PolyCystic Ovarian Syndrome (PCOS, more on that later) and working with thousands of women at my Manhattan-based FLO Living Center, that there's a formula for finding your FLO and for maintaining incredible hormonal health. Specifically, it's my five-step protocol, described in the chapters to come, which uses food therapeutically and changes lifestyle habits for improved health.

In this book, I teach you to incorporate specific medicinal foods to strengthen the health of the organs of hormone production and balance; help you embrace your exquisitely female self, energy, and life's purpose; and encourage you to connect with a like-minded community at FLOliving.com. I plan to address women in all stages of their reproductive health—i.e., their twenties, thirties, and forties—though the younger a woman starts, the better.

PCOS, premenstrual syndrome (PMS), fibroids, cystic ovaries, depression, thyroid issues, adrenal fatigue, irritable bowel syndrome (IBS), amenorrhea, dysmenorrhea, unexplained infertility, low libido, acne/rosacea/eczema, weight problems, human papillomavirus (HPV)—a lot of weighty medical terms to describe a lot of serious and challenging conditions. How can one protocol prevent and treat so many different "castaway conditions"? In WomanCode, I'll break down the answer in a way that's so simple, you won't remember a time when you didn't talk and think in your code. As you read, you'll learn what I discovered in the early years of my practice: that hormones seek balance and when you disrupt the endocrine system that governs them, you'll present with a symptom, then another, then another, until you have a condition. The conditions that women exhibit might be different from one female to the next, based on your genetic predisposition and lifestyle factors, but focusing on the symptoms and/or the conditions is less valuable than addressing the underlying causes. By going to the root cause of endocrine disruption and treating it properly, we can actually trigger the endocrine system to get itself into healing mode and start functioning the way it was intended. That's because there's an order and logic to how your endocrine system works. Once you gain a deeper understanding of how your hormones work, which won't remain a mystery much longer, you'll know what you need to do for your endocrine system to enable it to perform much better than it does today.

WomanCode will also serve as a touchstone for gynecologists, endocrinologists, and IVF specialists who want to "prescribe" the WomanCode method to patients as a complementary and integrative solution. To raise standard gynecological care, women and gynecologists must begin to collaborate where they can. I believe that medicine of the future is going to be a hybrid form—one in which people take greater responsibility for their own health instead of relying exclusively on doctors to make them better when they get sick. In this new hybrid, people will seek out a stronger understanding of how their bodies work and what they need to do to take care of themselves on a day-to-day basis. When medical issues arise, they can reach out to a team of wonderful practitioners in a variety of different specialties for guidance. Patients will know where they need to go to get the right information and won't expect one practitioner to have all the answers—and, most important, they'll know how to listen to their bodies to guide them toward finding the solutions they need.

I believe that this new relationship between gynecologists, patients, and FLO Living can change the paradigm of women's healthcare. Most women know very little about our hormonal bio-chemistry, and as a result, we're making choices about our menstrual care, fertility, and libido that have long-term negative repercussions. Among even the smartest women I know, Sex Ed was the first and last time they formally learned anything about their bodies, periods, and hormones; the rest has been picked up from magazines and friends.

I envision the new paradigm as a pyramid supporting each individual woman who sits on top benefiting from all that support while taking an active role in her healthcare. She visits her doctor regularly for exams, blood work, and checkups. Her doctor is open-minded to and supportive of all the ways in which she is experimenting with foods and supplements to feel her best. She is letting go of her passive relationship with her body because of all of the nutritional support and holistic health coaching she is receiving from FLOliving every day between her regular doctor visits. She's on top of her symptoms, on top of her nutrition and self-care, and on top of her health.

Finally, *WomanCode*'s mission isn't limited to making our endocrine systems sing. After working with hormonally imbalanced women for ten years, I've learned that getting healthy for health's sake is not a big enough game for us to play—at least, not for the long term. When you're healthy and feeling well, you have the energy to move in the direction of your dreams and to create the life you want to live. That's why I'm so passionate about helping women: when your endocrine system is working at its best, you're more excited about yourself and about life. This, in turn, leads you to attract greater opportunities, enjoy moments of creative expression, and connect more intimately with others. That's when you'll feel the fullness of your power, your life-force energy, and your fullest potential. *WomanCode*, the book, embodies the key elements of the WomanCode message and reveals a powerful solution to healing the silent epidemic of hormone imbalance. *WomanCode* offers the promise of a healthier, more vital, more inspiring tomorrow—one in which you can relate to your body in a new way and connect with your very best life.

I've had the privilege to bear witness to so many women using my approach and reclaiming their health. In the ten years since opening the FLO Living Center, I've worked with women on five continents; I've had a doctor call asking me what I had done to their patient so that an ovarian cyst that was operable completely disappeared; I've seen fibroids shrink, endometriosis kept at bay, anxiety and depression lift; I've watched women lose hundreds of pounds; I've seen so many women get pregnant after IVF failed; I've helped women transition off the Pill without having pre-Pill symptoms return; and I've helped women recover their energy and uncover their passion and purpose in life. I absolutely love my work and the women I get to work with and I'm so honored and excited that I get to share this process with you. This is my journey, it's your journey, and it's time for a new conversation and a fresh start for an area of women's health that has long been unappreciated.

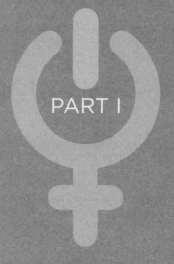

PART I

UNLOCKING YOUR WOMANCODE

CHAPTER 1

Putting an End to Your Suffering. Period.

I f you think your period is a burden, you're not alone. If you're worried about your fertility and it seems like many women around you are struggling to conceive, it's not all in your head. If you're in your twenties, thirties, or forties and your libido is MIA, you're not on your own either. If you navigate your day, your career, and your relationships with more head than heart, you've picked up the right book. If you've ever considered your female body to be messy and unruly, I'm about to change your mind about that. Because I'm here to tell you that your body is capable of so much more than pain, exhaustion, blame, and confusion. When you decode your own physiology, you're able to help your body heal and use that body to create the life you desire.

I know it may sound hard to believe from where you are right now—perhaps curled up with a heating pad, frustrated with dozens of self-empowerment books, waiting for your doctor to return your call(s), and fed up with procedures and drug therapies that have failed you. For the past ten years, I've run a successful holistic health practice in Manhattan that helps women rebalance their hormones and achieve astonishing levels of health and happiness. Women come to me with the core of their bodies broken. Their periods are irregular, they can't get pregnant, they're on a bunch of antidepressants and other meds, they have no sex drive or energy, they have no passion for their career, they don't know what their life's purpose is, and they're unhappy in their relationships.

Then, as we begin to work together, something takes place that's so extraordinary I've built my whole career on sharing it with others. When I invite these women to start learning about and observing their biology and hormones, I witness an incredible transformation in their entire being. Otherwise frustrated females fall in love with their hormones and bodily functions—the same ones that gave them cramps, cysts, and depression for years. And once these women begin to understand and restore their hormone balance with my protocol, they not only realize that their bodies are strong enough to heal themselves, but they learn how to use that power to become the fullest, most potent expression of themselves imaginable.

What these women have experienced and what I'm going to hand you are the keys to unlocking your very own WomanCode. At its most basic, your WomanCode is your endocrine system. It's the way your female body operates. To understand your WomanCode is to understand how your body works from a deeply functional level. When you have access to your code you're able to interpret all of the signs and symptoms your endocrine system is sending you. Only then can you make sense of your body and engage with it on a daily basis to create a natural state of hormonal health and balance. By far, the most extraordinary part of understanding your WomanCode is that it enables you to live in what I call the "FLO."

So what if I told you that if you really understood how your body works and made a few changes to your diet and lifestyle to create certain effects on your hormones, you too could find your FLO and have the energy, mental focus, and stable moods to live your best life? That you could run your business, have great relationships, and pursue as much fun and adventure as your stamina would allow? You'd be excited to give it a try, right? Well, it won't be long before you realize what my clients did: that taking care of your body—not just to get well, but *as a means to having the most fulfilling life you can have*—is one sweet deal. It's a matter of understanding how your body works, what the underlying causes of your hormonal issues are, and what you need to do daily to maintain hormonal balance. You're not out to achieve "perfect health," because that doesn't exist in nature and therefore makes no sense for your body. But I can help you commit to the science and education of how your body works, honor what it requires every meal, every day, and manage your relationship with your body by listening to its needs. Together, we'll help your body become the channel for your greatest dreams and pursuits.

So why should you trust me as your guide? I'm a holistic health coach. I use a functional nutrition approach to improve the function of body systems and organs with specific medicinal foods and my specialization is in women's reproductive endocrinology. I'd love for you to have faith in me and the life-changing WomanCode protocol I've developed because I've walked in your strappy sandals and have felt the frustration when there seems to be no solution available. I've done so much research, studying, and experimenting that I was able not only to heal my own body but also to help women with various hormonal conditions restore their well-being. No matter what you've been through up this point, I get it. But I also know, because of how your body, hormones, and endocrine system are designed to seek balance and heal, that you can access a whole new experience of your health and life when you take this journey with me.

I'd Like to Thank My Period

Based on how I spent my free time as a twelve-year-old, I probably could have guessed what my future career track would be. Every day after lunch I and my best friends Kristen, Katie, and Melissa barreled out the front doors of our elementary school to sneak over to a dividing wall at the side of the building. While the other students raced toward the fields for thirty minutes of recess, we chose to climb up and sit on top of a wall that didn't look too dangerous when you saw it head-on—but if you were sitting up top and glanced over your shoulder, at the side of the wall that faced away from the playground, you saw a serious twelve-foot-drop. Thinking back on that wall now, I realize how perfectly symbolic it was for us. During the spring of sixth grade, we were looking ahead to junior high, unavoidably perched on the precipice of pubescence. Most girls in school didn't seem fazed by the monumental event of menarche, but I was fascinated and excited to embrace my first signs of womanhood. I remember reading a neighbor's books while babysitting for her kids—namely, *What to Expect When You're Expecting* and *The Joy of Sex*. *Wow,* I'd think. *I'm so lucky that I get to have a woman's body. It does the coolest stuff!* I was always twelve going on thirty.

So "The Period Club," as I named it, gathered daily to discuss all the physical and emotional changes we were experiencing at the time (not to mention the usual social drama of tweendom). In psychic fashion I'd try to predict, in order, when each of my friends would get her period—who'd come first (Kristen), second (Katie), third (Melissa), and fourth (alas, me). Well, I should have bet my allowance, because that was precisely the order in which it went down. By the beginning of seventh grade, all three of my girlfriends had gotten their periods, but what I didn't know yet was that it would take until February of my sophomore year of high school—I would be fifteen at the time—to complete the prophecy and get my period, too. Nor did I know that the journey beginning back in sixth grade would soon guide the course of my entire life.

I credit my period with more than I imagine most people do. It has been my compass, has led me through my greatest challenges, has shown me the miracles of physical healing, has altered the course of my career, has introduced me to some really tremendous people, and has helped me understand and experience the power of feminine energy. In short, it's opened me up to a world that I never would have imagined for myself—and yes, I have my menstrual cycle to thank for it.

Everyone Has a Story—Here's Mine!

So if you can, picture me as I am now: five feet six, with thick and wavy brown hair, luminous skin, and a feminine, curvaceous 150 pounds. But let me tell you, I wasn't always this way.

As my friends developed "normally" during puberty, I was having a much less appealing experience: I was an androgynous, chubby, and acne-spotted child with thick, untamable hair. A young Audrey Hepburn, I wasn't. Once I finally got my first period, it came only two to four times a year. At first, I thought this was convenient—no maxi-pads under my leggings and all—but as I got older, my health and appearance began to need attention. Most doctors say standard procedure for a girl's first gynecology visit is after her first period, or as soon as she's sexually active. Since I was a late bloomer, I had to wait until my sixteenth birthday to see the gynecologist. During my first visit, and every one that followed, I always felt eager to discuss my feelings about my health—from weight gain, to pimples, to irregular periods, to sleep issues—because I always suspected that I wasn't 100 percent "right."

Yet the call-and-response with my docs was always the same, and always a major disappointment. I'd say, over and over again, that something was "off" with me, and whichever doctor I was seeing at the time would repeatedly insist that I go on birth control pills. I'd press her on how the pills would help me, and she'd just tell me to take the meds, appreciate the artificial cycle, and accept that "it will be better than nothing." It might sound bold to question a doctor this way, especially as a kid, but I come from a family that taught me to be wary of meds with no clear benefit, and never to accept when people were condescending to me because I was a child or woman. Besides, even to a teenager's ears, it didn't sound scientifically or medically sound to prescribe a course of treatment when the cause or condition hadn't been identified. So I'd defer taking the drug course and continue to spiral into poor health without answers. Then I'd see new doctors who'd tell me that I had an endocrine problem or maybe a slow thyroid. But all of their tests would come back inconclusive, and I'd be back where I started.

Eventually, my weight hit a high of two hundred pounds, I was covered in painful cystic acne on my face, chest, and back, and I got my period only twice a year. In college at Johns Hopkins, I spiraled into such a deep depression that during one semester I slept most of the day and looked for ways to escape my physical pain at night. I found myself vulnerable to the stereotypical collegiate binge drinking to numb how miserable I felt, tried to survive on one turkey sandwich a day to lose weight, downed copious amounts of caffeine to keep my energy up, and managed to fail a semester of Italian, even though I grew up speaking the romance language and aced every test I took. My Italian teacher gave me my first and only F because I didn't go to class—but the only reason I was a no-show was because my body literally couldn't function at 9 A.M. I'd reached a new low and was more afraid for my health than I had ever been, especially since none of my physicians knew what was going on.

So around the age of twenty, when I was still a college student, I decided to take matters into my own hands. Being the science nerd that I am, I went to the library and researched a bunch of medical journals to find out if I could help myself. Late one night, I ran across a brief article in an obstetrics journal about Stein-Leventhal disease— or what's now called polycystic ovarian syndrome (PCOS). As I read through the story, I was amazed at how perfectly I fit the classic presentation of the condition! I had chills. It was a bell-ringer of a moment.

The next morning, I marched myself into my latest gynecologist's office at Johns Hopkins, placed the article in front of her, and demanded that she give me what I learned was the only conclusive test for the condition—a transvaginal ultrasound. This painless procedure, in which a probe is used to look at a woman's reproductive organs, would be able to show if my ovaries were dotted with the cysts that give the condition its name. The doc was thrown off-guard by my bluntness but most graciously did the procedure then and there. Sure enough, my instincts were dead-on correct: there the cysts were, visible on the sonogram machine. Both ovaries were covered in multiple cysts. She and I were quiet for a minute as she cleaned me up and we moved from the exam room back to her office. Then we had the conversation that would change everything.

Even though I'd known in my gut that the sonogram would confirm my suspicions, I was *incredulous* that, despite having access to Harvard-trained gynecologists as a teen growing up in Newton, Massachusetts, and now as a student seeing a Johns Hopkins–trained gynecologist, no one had considered this diagnosis—or had even performed the very simple ultrasound to rule it out! Why hadn't anyone been able to piece together the puzzle of my various symptoms and test me for PCOS, given the compelling and rather startling statistic that says one out of eight women suffers with this condition? Why was this happening to me?

The bright side was that I'd finally diagnosed *myself* with a bona fide condition. But then I was hit with an even worse verdict: PCOS is considered incurable by Western medicine.

When No Is the Only Option

That grim verdict was given to me in pieces right after the ultrasound, when I asked my doctor what the prognosis for PCOS was. In a detached voice, she rattled off words that included diabetes, obesity, infertility, heart disease, and cancer. I breathed deeply—and as I did, I felt a resounding energy of *No!* rise up from the base of my spine and pour out of my every cell. Have you ever felt such a strong sense of conviction that it came from the deepest, wisest place inside you—a place you maybe never even knew was there? For me, this *No!* was that kind of mandate, a decision, a sum of my being . . . a sign that I needed to fight for my body. I asked what the recommended course of therapy might be, and the doctor advised hormone replacement therapy in the form of birth control pills. She said that I could go on Clomid when it came time to conceive, or have in-vitro fertilization (IVF) if necessary. As if I hadn't been pummeled enough, she added that I should probably consider other meds to control symptoms, such as Glucophage for insulin issues, Aldactone for hirsutism issues, Accutane for skin issues, and eventually blood pressure medication, and, and, and . . .

I was thrumming with this same *No!*—only it was louder and more determined now—and I thought I might actually start to levitate from the chair, so fast and furious was the vibration within me. Very calmly, I asked her a final question: Are there any *other* known ways to treat this?

My doctor's response was short and uninterested. Not to her knowledge, she said. That's when my foundation really began to crack—not only because I was thrown by my diagnosis, but also because I'd been planning to become an ob-gyn, and I assumed that when it came to healing the human body, medicine was the ultimate vehicle. Yet sitting in this office, I saw my doctor for the first time not just as a healer, but also as a person. And this person hadn't been trained to correctly examine my symptoms. Frankly, she didn't appear to know much more than what I'd garnered from my reading the night before. Though I wasn't really angry with her, I felt that I was on my own with this condition. In that moment, not only was I clear that I would have to rely on myself to find a solution, but I also recognized that pursuing a medical degree no longer felt like the right fit for me. Without realizing it at the time, over those past few years, as I'd struggled to understand what was wrong with me, I'd become much more interested in what I would later understand as functional medicine—a holistic approach to addressing the underlying causes of disease instead of treating the symptoms—than I was in traditional medicine.

I politely told my doctor that instead of taking her advice, I'd dedicate myself to researching other options for my healing and care. She tried to deter me, repeating stats about infertility and cancer, and insisted I should begin birth control that day. I'd be lying if I didn't admit that I was nervous to stand my ground, but that *No!* energy kept me from giving in. Again, I insisted I would heal the condition myself, and she smiled at me—out of either concern or frustration, I'm not sure which—and asked me to come see her after my healing journey was through. As much as we didn't see eye to eye on my situation, I'm eternally grateful to her and that conversation for kicking me out of the nest, out of my passive relationship with my body, and into my future.

So I buckled down, and when library research led to dead ends, I turned to real life. My talented esthetician, an angelic woman from my hometown, led me to the next clue. I visited her on school breaks to allow her loving hands to comfort my horrible skin. She did these really amazing facials. She was a Dr. Hauschka–trained professional who specialized in natural skin care and tried to help my acne. I told her about my recent diagnosis, and she offered to connect me with a colleague, a naturopathic doctor nearby. Maybe he could provide some insight?

This was excellent news to me and would most definitely usher in the next phase of my research process. I remember our meetings: this naturopath was convinced that my issues stemmed from an overgrowth of candida and proceeded to create a food and supplement regimen to address this. At that point, I realized and accepted that I'd have to double as both guinea pig and investigative researcher to find out if there was a way to heal my body. But better to do so via natural means than chemical ones, I thought. So I agreed to work with him. I was on a mission, and there was no looking back.

For the next three years, I apprenticed with this doctor and others, experimenting with their techniques. In addition to the naturopath, I tracked down and began working with herbalists, acupuncturists, acupressure specialists, homeopaths—anyone that I felt had some perspective to offer. At one point, I followed a primarily carrot juice diet that turned my skin orange, yet this guinea pig kept going. I was willing to work with anyone and do anything to generate a change in my condition. I learned a lot during this time, but most of all, I learned that I was no closer to finding a solution than I'd been before.

The Discovery That Changed It All

My symptoms were still the same: I was carrying extra weight, I felt exhausted, I wasn't menstruating other than twice per year, my skin was covered in acne, and I was still searching for answers. I decided to go back to what I did best—researching—instead of endlessly trying cocktails of supplements and herbs to no avail. I vowed that I would do whatever was necessary to understand what had gone wrong in my endocrine system so that I could learn what I needed to do to correct it. I spent a lot of time studying endocrinology and the functions of my hormones, but I discovered that other fields had a great deal to teach me, too. These included Traditional Chinese Medicine (TCM), functional nutrition, and chronobiology.

TCM provided a framework for understanding the interconnectedness of glands and organs in the body in ways endocrinology could not. If there's a deficiency in one gland or organ, I learned, another will step in and overcompensate. This perspective allowed me to see the domino effect that can occur in the body: consistently poor diet or lifestyle choices can set off a chain reaction, and if you don't correct those choices, your endocrine system is forced to work in ways it shouldn't. This inevitably results in hormonal breakdown and causes the variety of symptoms that may have led you to pick up this book in the first place. While these first two fields—endocrinology and TCM—enabled me to understand how the endocrine system works, the question remained, How best to fix it? That's where the functional nutrition piece came in. In my research, I came to see just how powerfully impactful food could be, not only in resolving symptoms in the short term, but in helping the body stay symptom-free in the long term. If poor food choices could lead to a state of hormonal collapse, then well-chosen foods contained the nutrients necessary to support hormonal health. Through my research and personal experimentation, it became clear that food would be the key "medicine" to be used in my protocol.

My desire to learn even more about the endocrine system eventually led me to study chronobiology, which teaches that every system of the body has its own routine. Look no further than the menstrual cycle to see how beautifully the body works on a set schedule. Under ideal circumstances, there's a predictable ratio of hormones that happens four times per month, creating four distinct phases of the cycle. Similarly, each of our organs functions according to a chronobiological rhythm. The fact that blood pressure is higher in the morning and lower in the evening is a great example of chronobiology. Given these physiological routines, I couldn't help but think about how wonderful it would be if we could support each of the phases of the menstrual cycle with diet and lifestyle behaviors.

In time, my protocol grew from meshing these four fields. From endocrinology and TCM, I came to see that if you're not aware of certain choices you're making every single day, you can move yourself in a direction of hormonal breakdown more easily than you can imagine. Meanwhile, chronobiology teaches us that there's a rhythm and routine to how your body, including your hormones, works. And from functional nutrition, I learned that certain foods affect the health of specific organs, and micronutrients influence the release and elimination of certain hormones. I gathered this multifaceted information together to create a tool women could use to make the best choices for their reproductive and overall health every single day. It was a formula that none of my doctors had prescribed, something I'd never read about, and the start of a program that was proving itself in real time, in my body.

After nine months of implementing my protocol, over sixty pounds had melted away, my skin had cleared so exquisitely that strangers commented on its radiance, my depression had lifted, my moods had stabilized, and I had begun to ovulate and menstruate monthly.

Taking My Protocol to Other Women

Around this same time I got a job in Manhattan working as a marketing director for an online startup. I needed to support myself while taking the next step in following my passion: earning a degree from the Institute for Integrative Nutrition, then affiliated with Columbia University's Teachers College. A decade ago, my friends and family thought I'd lost my mind—health coaching, what on earth is that?—but my instincts about this discipline were spot on.

Health coaching was born nearly two decades ago. At the time, there was one main program—the Institute for Integrative Nutrition. These days, prestigious institutions like Duke University certify health coaches, and well-known physicians such as Dr. Mehmet Oz and Dr. Andrew Weil support our growing discipline. Holistic health coaches guide people to make diet and lifestyle changes in a sustainable way—that is, in a way that will still work for them decades down the road. We look at what people have been eating and doing that has created their symptoms and then work with them to develop a plan to resolve those problems. My greatest goal as a health coach is to guide patients to a point where they can bear witness to their own healing power. When a patient has attained his or her health goals and thanks me, I always tell them that if I did my job correctly, *I* was their best guide. *They*, however, did all of the essential work making the food and lifestyle shifts. I simply showed them how to think about their daily habits differently so they could heal themselves.

Today, the emerging health-coach trend reminds me of how chiropractors and acupuncturists were considered fringe thirty years ago, and now the benefits of engaging these methods is so well documented that most health insurance companies cover visits to such practitioners. Similarly, in the past ten years, we've started to see health coaches incorporated into corporate wellness programs and available for consultations at many doctors' offices, and these professionals are certified not only through accredited institutions but also through the American Association of Drugless Practitioners.

What's more, just as medicine has become more specialized over the years, health coaching is evolving into specific concentrations. Through core training and continuing education experience, there are health coaches who focus on diabetes control, cardiovascular issues, digestive disorders, and other specialties. That's exactly what I've done: because of my history and what I felt passionate about long before I discovered this as a career possibility, I've narrowed my focus within the field so that I can provide the most comprehensive care possible for helping patients overcome hormonally based gynecological issues.

As you can imagine, word got out through teachers and friends that I'd managed to heal myself from PCOS. I began seeing clients, a few at first, then a dozen, and then more than I could handle given my schedule and workload—so I quit my job. Initially, I wanted to work only with women who'd suffered, like me, with PCOS. Soon, though, my clients were telling their friends with PMS, fibroids, postpartum issues, and other hormone-based conditions about their experience. These women wanted, as I had, to help themselves without drugs or surgery; they needed a daily plan to manage the monthly cycle of suffering. They wanted to shrink their fibroids, get rid of their cysts, eliminate PMS, get pregnant, and/or rediscover their sex drive. I welcomed all of these women with the understanding that we'd apply my techniques to their situation and see what we discovered together. For the first time since my journey began, I wasn't alone anymore.

In those early years of my practice, I realized something very critical—that the underlying causes of hormonal imbalance are very similar, regardless of the symptoms. As a result, my protocol was, and continues to be, effective for most conditions related to the endocrine system. Out of all of this experimentation came an under-standing of what the true underlying causes of hormonal imbalance are, which was followed by the discovery of what became my five-step healing protocol.

Heal Your Hormones, Improve Your Life

Often, when I first meet with clients, they want me to tell them how to "fix" their body. Well, if there's one thing I'd love for you to take away from this book, it's that you can't *fix* a hormonal issue. And yet clients always feel healthier and happier after completing my program. That's because I help them understand a pearl of wisdom that I'm now going to share with you: the only way your hormones can achieve balance is if your *body* does the job—and *only* if you safeguard and nurture it, with every meal and habit, every day, to optimize endocrine function.

This book and my five-step protocol will address your underlying hormonal issues so that you can experience immediate improve-ments in whatever condition you're coping with today. In the long run, adopting the protocol will help you stay healthy, avoid future hormonal breakdown, preserve your fertility, protect your libido, and extend your youthfulness. Soon this experience of health and vitality will become a foundation from which you'll be able to create a life around your deepest passions and desires. And with the protocol, you'll be able to trust that your body will always be there for you, to support you through the process of designing your very best life. Ultimately, I've dedicated my life and career to women's hormonal health because I believe wholeheartedly that when you live in part-nership with your body, you have access to an innate power to create positive change in your life and the world around you.

The WomanCode Five-Step Protocol

My five-step protocol is designed, in the sequence outlined below, to address the underlying causes of hormonal problems and to support the essential functions of your endocrine system so your hormones can work in a healthy, balanced way. Think of these steps as the keys to unlocking your WomanCode:

Stabilize your blood sugar

Nurture your adrenal glands

Support your organs of elimination

Syncing with your menstrual cycle

Engage your feminine energy

Chapter 2 will look at the underlying causes of hormonal imbalances. Chapter 3 will introduce you to your endocrine system as a whole and teach you the secrets of your WomanCode. Chapter 4 will take you through the first three steps of the protocol and help you get in the FLO. Chapters 5 and 6 will focus on the fourth step. Chapters 7 and 8 will give additional support for fertility and libido concerns. Chapters 9 and 10 will focus on the fifth step of the protocol.

Before I explain what these steps mean and how to do them, I want to urge you to please start at the beginning and complete each step along the way. This is a *cumulative* protocol: each step builds on the one before it. How soon can you expect to start seeing results? In my experience, women who truly commit to the first step and stabilize their blood sugar start to feel a dramatic difference in their well-being within the second week. As you begin to deeply improve the way the endocrine system is operating through the protocol, you can expect to see improvements in menstruation, fertility, and libido within two to four months. Yet the real value of this protocol for your health, your hormones, and your life is not as a short-term fix, but as a new way of living. It proposes a new way of operating and caring for your body in order to protect your delicate hormonal balance for years to come.

One-on-One with Alisa

Throughout the book I want you to feel as if you're sitting down with me at my FLO Living Center in personal one-on-one health-coaching sessions. In these sessions I will guide you to think about what you've learned in a constructive, digestible, and individual way. I will also give you assignments to address any underlying behavioral, emotional, or thought patterns that could prevent those changes from taking root and will encourage you to start thinking about how you will implement these changes into your life in ways that are authentic and practical for you.

What's Your Story?

Do you *believe* that your body can transform into a healthy state? If you don't, why not? What's the story running around in your mind? I want to help you recognize that you may have a very powerful script in your head—one telling you that change isn't possible, even as you're attempting to embark on change. If this is true for you, I want to make sure you're aware of these negative thoughts and bring them from the unconscious to the conscious, where they can be examined and reshaped. Then, every time you start to engage part of the protocol and hear the negative script spring into action, you can begin to replace the old script with a new one. Use plenty of positive assurances: *I am healing. Change is possible. I am getting better. My body is capable of fixing itself.* The more you bring positive statements to mind, the faster you'll interrupt the negativity, until it's no longer your first reaction—or any reaction—when you set out to create change in your body and health.

Is the WomanCode Protocol Right for Me?

This protocol addresses three primary goals: period perfection, fertility preservation and enhancement, and libido restoration and improvement. If you identify with any of the bullet points below, you've picked up the right book.

Period Perfection

Are you plagued by any of the following?

- Fibroids
- Premenstrual syndrome
- Premenstrual dysphoric disorder
- Polycystic ovary syndrome
- Ovarian cysts
- Endometriosis
- Heavy periods
- Missing periods
- Irregular cycles
- Cystic breasts

Fertility Preservation and Enhancement

Do you see yourself in any of these statements?

- I want to conceive naturally.
- I haven't been able to conceive, and there's no medical explanation why.
- I tried IVF and it didn't work (or I have to take a break from it).
- I'd like to use a natural, food-based solution to prepare my body for my IVF cycle.
- I've experienced multiple miscarriages.
- I'm a single twenty- or thirty-something, but I want to conceive easily when the time is right for me.
- I have a beautiful baby . . . and now I also have postpartum depression (PPD).
- No matter what I do, I can't shed the baby weight.

Libido Restoration and Improvement

Do any of these symptoms sound familiar?
- Fatigue/exhaustion
- Insomnia
- Depression
- Fuzzy-headedness
- Thyroid issues such as hypothyroidism or hyperthyroidism
- Anxiety
- Mood swings
- Lack of sexual thoughts
- Low sex drive/desire
- Inability to reach orgasm or attain the sensations you once had during orgasm
- Difficult perimenopause or menopause

What About Complementary and Alternative Medicine (CAM)?

CAM therapies can be tremendously helpful when the right treatments are used for the right reasons. But it's important to maintain realistic expectations: these treatments provide excellent symptom support, but it's food that is able to generate the deep changes needed to create speedy improvement of your condition. They can, and often do, fit nicely with the deeper transformation involved in the WomanCode protocol, but in my experience with clients they won't bring about hormonal health on their own. While the protocol focuses on healing underlying hormonal issues, CAM therapies can be very helpful complements to the nutritional work of WomanCode.

I use CAM treatments in my own life on a monthly or quarterly basis to help keep my body humming along nicely. They're my go-to treatments when I want to turn up the volume on my self-care, or when I need to de-stress more deeply than my current routines allow me to. I've had sessions with every single type of practitioner in the chart below. If you're curious whether any of these therapies could help you, check out the chart to see my recommendations for how and when to use them based on the category of issue—menstrual, fertility, or libido—you're experiencing.

CAM Therapy	Menstrual	Fertility	Energy/Libido
Acupuncture	Acupuncture is great for improving blood flow to reproductive organs, which can be useful if you experience heavy periods with lots of clotting or very light, barely-there periods.	In addition to improving circulation to the reproductive organs, a skilled acupuncturist will target the energy channels associated with conception.	During acupuncture, you experience a really powerful cortisol flush, which removes the stress hormone that may be interfering with your energy and libido. Your acupuncturist may also target the adrenals and other major energy points during your sessions.

CAM Therapy	Menstrual	Fertility	Energy/Libido
Massage	Look for a licensed practitioner who offers Maya abdominal massage, a noninvasive, external technique designed to guide the reproductive organs into their proper position. This aids their function and releases physical and emotional blockages to restore health to the uterus and surrounding organs. If you experience severe menstrual cramps, ask the practitioner to show you techniques you can perform on your own.	Maya abdominal massage or Clear Passage Technique can also be helpful if you experience fertility issues due to scarring or other structural issues/ blockages. It can help improve the health of the uterus so you may have a greater likelihood of being able to maintain a pregnancy.	Regular, traditional massage in a soothing environment can help you relax and enjoy your experience in your body. Avoid intense muscular massage, such as shiatsu, which can trigger the stress response; instead, look for gentle, deep-tissue, or Swedish techniques.
Naturopathy	A naturopath can help address nutrient deficiency issues such as anemia, or use supplementation to spot-treat symptoms associated with PMS such as depression and anxiety.	A naturopath may do a thirty-day saliva test of hormonal fluctuations to find out whether your hormonal ratios during your cycle are optimal for conceiving. This is a great place to start to make sure your hormones are working appropriately— and to try to correct them naturally if they're not—before seeking medical intervention to conceive.	A customized supplementation program, based on the causes of your lack of energy and/or lack of libido, may help.

CAM Therapy	**Menstrual**	**Fertility**	**Energy/Libido**
Applied kinesiology	A practitioner can help find out whether you have allergies you don't know about that may be making your symptoms worse and work with you to remove those foods to help improve your cycle.	If you're having difficulty conceiving, an applied kinesiologist will do a systemic investigation of what might be going on energetically that could pose challenges in conceiving, and work with you to correct it.	In addition to checking for allergies that could be sucking your energy, an applied kinesiologist can perform energy-clearing techniques to help you feel more open and relaxed.
Chiropractic treatment	Proper alignment of the hips, sacrum, pubic bones, and spine can increase proper circulation and function of the reproductive organs for easier periods.	Making sure the body is in optimal alignment and functioning without any structural interference can aid conception.	Improved alignment of the spine allows signals from the brain to flow more easily to all parts of your body, thus boosting energy and sexual response.
Herbalism	Specific herbs can be prescribed to help manage cramps, heavy or light flow, and even support regular ovulation.	Various herbs are known to support uterine health, which can support successful implantation.	Again, herbs here can be a valuable tool in helping to mitigate the effects of stress on adrenal health, which is at the source of healthy energy and libido.

CHAPTER 2

When Bad Hormones Happen to Good Women

New research from the National Institutes of Health confirms that a woman's menstrual health acts as a gauge of her vitality and overall health throughout her life. It's no surprise, then, that some of my patients with chronic symptoms were well on their way to obesity, diabetes, hypertension, heart disease, infertility, premature aging, and gallbladder disease when they first walked through my door. If this latest data holds fast, it further affirms why we need to try our best to be vigilant about healing our bodies, especially considering how many "lady parts" are in trouble:

- Over twenty million women suffer from polycystic ovary syndrome (PCOS), fibroids, endometriosis, painful/difficult/heavy periods, and thyroid and adrenal issues.

- More specifically, one in nine women suffers from PCOS.

- Fibroids occur in three out of every ten women over the age of thirty-five, though women in their twenties can have them, too.
- About one in ten, or over eight million, U.S. women have endometriosis (176 million globally).
- Thirteen million Americans have underactive thyroid function, only half of whom have been correctly diagnosed. Women are five times more likely than men to be diagnosed with hypothyroidism.
- One in eight couples is infertile.
- Fibrocystic breasts affect 20 to 40 percent of menstruating women.
- An estimated seven million women meet the diagnostic criteria for clinical depression.
- Every ten minutes, twelve hysterectomies are performed in the United States—that's six hundred thousand every year!

Crazy? Yes. The assumption that most women don't know about or talk about this stuff? Scary. The fact that there are no natural solutions in place to help us recover? Unacceptable. That's the very reason why I earlier referred to these hormonal issues as "castaway conditions." There's only so much that Western medicine has to offer besides extreme interventions—such as surgery—when you're in great distress. When your situation is less extreme, you might find yourself leaving visit after visit feeling hopeless and discouraged. But with all of the advances in functional medicine today, there's so much each of us can be doing that we no longer need to feel cast away. I'll show you how to take the reins of your health, explain how the body works, and teach you what you need to do to heal forever.

What in the Panties Is Going On?

For the past decade I've dedicated myself to helping women improve their health in three core categories of hormonally based gynecological issues: menstruation, fertility, and libido. These essential categories determine the quality of a woman's health overall and either enhance or impede her FLO—in other words, how vital she feels depends on how well those three systems are operating.

Up to 40 percent of all women who've been diagnosed with low sexual desire also report depression. And for those on antidepressants, as many as 50 percent experience a decrease in desire.

During these same ten years, I've also identified four of the greatest obstacles women face to living with the best possible hormonal health. I call them "FLO Blockers" because, from a biological perspective, they all serve as endocrine disruptors in one way or another. In part II, I will explain how you can clear a natural path through this toxic landscape, but for now let's examine what's holding you back from feeling, doing, and being your very best.

FLO Blocker 1: Misinformation about your hormones

Few women understand how their bodies function, so most don't know how to make informed decisions about how to treat hormones when they're on the fritz. Many women spend lots of time researching their symptoms online, yet have no proper knowledge of how to take care of themselves in a way that will avoid hormonal collapse. If I asked you to draw a chart of the hormones involved in menstruation over a thirty-day period, could you do it . . . *and* explain it to me? No? Well, please don't feel badly about this. In ten years of my practice, I've never met a woman who could sketch this out for me, which leads to my bigger point: when you're not properly taught this information, you simply can't make *informed* decisions about what ails you when the problem is hormone-related. Furthermore, when you don't know how things work and have the misunderstanding that hormones are illogical, erratic, and chaotic, you can't even believe that your body is *capable* of performing any better. As a result, many women fall into the trap of believing that suffering is an inevitable part of being born with a female body. It's no wonder, then, that misinformation has become an enormous FLO Blocker in women's lives today and has put hormonal health on the line for millions of women.

FLO Blocker 2: Cultural conditioning

I also like to call this category "hypersuck," because women tend to get "sucked" into believing that our bodies are wild, scary, shameful places that need to be managed by an outside source, medicated, controlled, and sterilized. (We have the media and other social influences to thank for that.) We are rewarded for acting/speaking/looking like young girls versus confident women. We have too few powerful, healthy role models, but plenty of exhausted moms and emaciated models front and center on our cultural stage. We have a hard time appreciating our grown-up female bodies. We're made to feel that female intuition is fickle. We suspect that our energy is unstable. We're conditioned to think that our periods are shameful and disgusting. We look for ways to fix what's broken. We discipline the highs and lows of our female essence. We disconnect from our own bodies and, often, our deepest sense of knowing. Ultimately, our mind-body conversation tips the scales in a negative direction, and this too affects hormone balance. And since hypersuck (that old cultural conditioning) tricks us into thinking our bodies are *supposed* to be acting this way, we allow serious hormonal issues—and all the symptoms that tag along—to linger for years before seeking out any kind of sustainable action to help ourselves heal. Sadly, many women lose faith long before reaching the point of action.

FLO Blocker 3: Our toxic environment and lifestyle

Exposure to endocrine disruptors (chemicals that interfere with the production, release, transport, metabolism, or elimination of the body's natural hormones) can occur through air, water, soil, food, and consumer products. These disruptors can mimic naturally occurring hormones, potentially causing overproduction and underproduction of actual hormones. They block the way natural hormones and their receptors are made or controlled. Some of the dirtiest culprits include dry-cleaning chemicals, skin-care products, and pesticides. Chemical compounds known as xenoestrogens—including industrial compounds such as polychlorinated biphenyl (PCB), bisphenol A (BPA), and phthalates—are at an all-time high. These xenoestrogens have estrogenic-like effects on living organisms. It's no coincidence, given all the estrogenic chemicals in our lakes and seas, that there are fewer male fish in the world; in the human world, men produce less than half as many sperm as they did fifty years ago, and women suffer from estrogen-dependent diseases such as endometriosis at a historically high rate. We're also inundated by stress, another endocrine disruptor. Chronic low-grade anxiety affects the feedback between your brain's hypothalamus, pituitary gland, and adrenal glands—a configuration known as the HPA-axis, which regulates digestion, immunity, moods, libido, and energy.

FLO Blocker 4: Our modern diet and the desire for quick-fix solutions to heal our bodies

This FLO Blocker is a twofold issue. First, we're exposed to conflicting and confusing information about what to eat (think: fads such as no-carb diets, low-fat diets, all-juice cleanses, fasting, and more.) We try our best to be "healthy" but inevitably consume too many carbs, too little fat, too few nutrients, too much sugar, and too much alcohol and caffeine. Your entire endocrine system relies on the micronutrients you consume in your diet, so when these levels fall short, your hormones are thrown for a loop and your reproductive health suffers.

••

Organic Food—How Much Is Enough?

There's a lot of confusion about how much of an impact eating organic has on our health. A recent study by Stanford University showed that in fact the nutritional values of organic foods are nearly identical to those that are commercially produced (with pesticides). Of course this makes sense: an apple is an apple and broccoli is broccoli no matter how you grow it, and it is extremely logical that the nutrient content—calories and vitamin content—would be the same. However, what is most definitely not the same is what you're getting in addition to that commercially grown apple or broccoli that you're eating. These foods contain pesticides, organophosphates, and other farming chemicals that wreak havoc on your delicate endocrine system, congesting your liver, acting like estrogen in your body (often referred to as xenoestrogens), and confusing the hormonal conversation your body needs to have to create balance and avoid symptoms and diseases. Now, all of this is enough to make anyone a bit anxious, and I've seen women, as well as myself when I first got started, develop a type of eating disorder called "orthorexia," a term meaning hyper-correct/ clean eating. This is behavior where a woman will only eat foods, and will delay

In addition, chemicals in foods—antibiotics, added hormones, insecticides, and more—can jeopardize your hormonal balance.

The second problem with this FLO Blocker is that it has us over-relying on medications to fix our health instead of taking responsibility for healing ourselves. How many of you have heard the expression, "Take two of these and call me in the morning"? This seemingly harmless cliché sums up how passively many of us relate to our bodies and illustrates how much we rely on taking a little something to fix a big problem. To tackle this FLO Blocker, in later chapters I'm going to show you how certain foods serve as medicine for your endocrine system, and for specific symptoms as well.

eating until she is able to eat foods, that she feels are correct and safe—for orthorexics typically this means organic foods. The great news here is that when following the WomanCode protocol for 80 percent or more of the time, your endocrine system will be well supported for and better able to handle the 20 percent or fewer times that you're eating somewhat off protocol in terms of organic foods. Some foods are more offensive than others when it comes to chemicals. Here is a list of organic food must-haves for your shopping reference.

WomanCode Organic Food Essentials

- **Fruits:** blueberries, strawberries, apples, melons, pears, peaches
- **Miscellaneous:** celery, peppers, tomatoes
- **Root vegetables:** potatoes, sweet potatoes, squash
- **Leafy green vegetables:** all lettuces, kale, cabbage, spinach, other greens
- **Animal protein:** beef, poultry, dairy, eggs (especially because these animals, when not organically fed and properly pastured, are fed a diet of antibiotics, growth hormones, and genetically modified foods that will exacerbate your existing hormonal imbalance)

With so many FLO Blockers on the loose, more women than ever are hormonally sensitive and susceptible to imbalances. Recognizing these impediments is an essential step toward your most vital health. And if you read between the lines, you'll notice that all of these FLO Blockers are examples of ways our society strives for perfection—with model bodies, perfect careers, idyllic families, packaged foods, and quick fixes. If this sounds all too familiar and exhausting, you can exhale now. WomanCode is not about having the perfect life; rather, it's about nurturing your body to help you have a life that's authentic and fulfilling for you.

I Couldn't Make This Stuff Up

No FLO Blocker plays nice, but some of the most hazardous FLO Blockers reside in your makeup bag. This particularly stinks because a recent study in the United Kingdom found that women who use makeup absorb almost five pounds of chemicals into their bodies each year! What's more, cosmetic products aren't subject to FDA approval, so it's up to you to read labels if you want to protect your hormones.

In the name of cleaning out your beauty bag, here are a few personal-care items with the most offending endocrine disruptors. When it's time to shop for replacements, check out the appendix titled "WomanCode-Approved Products" for health-safe suggestions.

- **Reconsider your:** nail polish, body lotion, and deodorant
- **Toss if the label lists:** chemicals from the phthalate family (DBP, DEHP)
- **Why endocrine disruptors are used in the first place:** to make products soft and malleable

- **Reconsider your:** toothpaste, shampoo, bath salts, and body/shower gel
- **Toss if the label lists:** sodium lauryl sulfate (SLS) or sodium lauryl ether sulfate (SLES)

Every Woman Is Different

Right about now, you may be wondering why *you* have different symptoms or conditions than your sister or best friend when every woman's endocrine system functions the same way and we're all victims of these same FLO Blockers. There's actually a very simple biological answer for this.

Though we're all exposed to endocrine system disruptors, the conditions that women develop vary from one woman to the next based on genetic predispositions and lifestyle factors. Everyone's

- *Why these endocrine disruptors are used in the first place:* as agents and emulsifiers

- *Reconsider your:* conditioner, foundation, concealer, facial mask, and skin cream
- *Toss if the label lists:* chemicals known as parabens (including methyl, propyl, butyl, and ethyl)
- *Why these endocrine disruptors are used in the first place:* as germicides and preservatives

- *Reconsider your:* soap, hairspray, eyeliner, talc, shaving cream, and hair spray
- *Toss if the label lists:* chemicals from the anolamine family (DEA, TEA, MEA)
- *Why these endocrine disruptors are used in the first place:* as emulsifiers, pH adjusters, preservatives, foaming agents

- *Reconsider your:* petroleum jelly and skin and lip products
- *Toss if the label lists:* petrolatum
- *Why this endocrine disruptor is used in the first place:* as a moisturizer

cells, glands, and organs function similarly, but genetics plays a big part in how well those components do their jobs. Just as your muscles are wrapped onto your skeleton by a layer of collagen, there is a thin layer of protein that wraps around your DNA strands. Based on environmental factors like diet, stress, and prenatal nutrition, that protein either constricts or expands around certain genes, turning them off or on. This process is the subject of a new field of research called epigenetics, which grew out of the human genome project. At its most basic, epigenetics is the study of changes in gene expression that are affected almost exclusively by diet and lifestyle factors. Recent findings from studies at Duke University and Groningen University in the Netherlands show that how you eat and live actually gets passed down to at least one successive generation through this epigenetic process. One recent study by scientists in the Netherlands found that the diet of human adults causes changes in all cells—including sperm and egg cells—that can be passed on to offspring and continue for generations. Another study found that overfed mouse pups developed signs of metabolic syndrome (insulin resistance, obesity, and glucose intolerance) and passed some of these traits to future generations, which showed symptoms of metabolic syndrome even if they didn't overeat.

In a study among overweight adults put on a diet, sleep, a lifestyle factor, turned out to be a determinant of success: subjects who slept an average of five hours and fifteen minutes per night lost less body fat than those who slept an average of seven hours and twenty-five minutes per night.

So if your friend isn't predisposed to PCOS, she can eat more fast food without suffering from weight gain and cystic acne than you can if you carry this genetic predisposition. And even within your own family, genes are expressed in different ways; although your sister didn't struggle with infertility, for example, you still may. In addition to this genetic component, your friend and sister may have avoided more endocrine-disrupting chemicals and foods than you did, and/or their bodies may have managed to temper the effects of those chemicals more effectively than yours.

Now for the exciting part! Epigenetically speaking, if you eat to support your beautiful hormones, your body won't keep manifesting your symptoms. That's the wonder of epigenetic and nutritional genomic research. It provides hope that you can have real control over your body from the inside out. In addition, scientists have determined that it takes on average seven years for your cells to regenerate, which is great news where you and your well-being are concerned, because it means that what you eat and do today will directly dictate the future quality of your health. Since on a cellular level you're a new person every seven years, the genetic material manufactured from that cell turnover sets you up for a future of thriving or nose-diving. All the more reason to make important changes now while you have plenty of years to look forward to enjoying a healthy body!

Every woman who picks up this book is coming to it from a different place and with a different purpose. That's what I love about working with women every single day—we're so hungry to squeeze more out of life, to reach a higher state of health, to create more, and to become our best selves. So whether you're looking for a little fine-tuning or are up to your chandelier earrings in hormonal symptoms, there's abundant information here for you. And you might have more in common with one another than you think. While some signs of hormonal imbalance, such as cramps or fibroids, seem obviously linked to a wonky endocrine system, clients are often surprised to learn that symptoms like insomnia and dandruff are hormonally based as well. You might feel generally healthy but experience the occasional headache or bout of constipation from time to time. What you may not realize is that these effects, too, are often due to glitches in your endocrine system or to habits (such as staying up all night or skipping meals) that can mess with your hormones and result in bothersome symptoms.

In order to know that you've reached certain health-improving checkpoints along the way throughout this journey, it's important to know where you're starting from today.

Below is a health assessment unlike any you've ever taken before. You'll see things in this assessment that you've never thought of as being hormonally based, but they're all connected and cumulatively representative of how well your endocrine system is performing. Taking this simple assessment will give you a picture of your endocrine function at this moment. Consider this your baseline—the starting point from which you'll build and improve your hormonal health.

....

Be in the Know: What Is WomanCode and FLO?

WomanCode is a system that balances female hormones, prevents menstrual troubles, and improves fertility and libido.

FLO is a lifestyle that is in sync with your unique biochemistry and is the state from which you powerfully create your life.

....

Decode Your Hormonal Clues

Ready for your first exercise on the road to having easier periods, enhanced fertility, more energy, and a hotter sex life? What I'd like for you to do now is circle the words below that relate to you and your body, and then earmark this page for later. We'll come back to it when it's time to put these clues into the bigger context of your general and reproductive health.

Metabolism and Stress Symptoms

- Carb cravings/binging
- Sugar and chocolate cravings
- Reliance on coffee, soda, and energy drinks
- Consuming more than three alcohol-based drinks per week
- Skipping meals
- Anxiety
- Insomnia
- Waking up during sleep
- Headaches
- Low libido
- Facial/body hair
- Weight gain
- Hypothyroidism
- Metabolic syndrome
- Diabetes

Elimination Symptoms

- Irritable bowel syndrome
- Oily skin
- Bloating and water retention
- Acne or cystic acne
- Dandruff
- Eczema
- Hair loss
- Constipation
- Diarrhea or loose stools
- Body odor
- Night sweats

Cycle Symptoms

- Mood swings
- PMS
- Irregular cycles
- Fibroids
- Ovarian Cysts
- Cystic breasts
- Breast tenderness
- Polycystic Ovarian Syndrome (PCOS)
- Unexplained infertility
- Cramps
- Heavy periods
- Painful periods
- Missing periods
- Migraines
- Depression

Discover Your Biological Blueprint

In this chapter you've learned about various factors in your body, life, and environment that threaten to put your lady parts at risk. So the question is, How can you create a life that puts your endocrine function first so that you can thrive in a world that's not designed to support your best endocrine health? You've come to the right place.

The first essential piece is to understand what your endocrine system is and how it works. This knowledge will chip away at FLO Blocker 1: misinformation about your hormones. Once you see what your hormones can and should do and internalize how this information relates to your uniquely female body, you'll take major leaps in the direction of building a life of hormonal balance. On a moment-to-moment basis, you'll be able to determine quickly which choices support your hormones and which threaten them. The next significant shift you'll make is moving from a passive to an active relationship with your body—literally partnering with your body to follow through with making those choices that keep you feeling your absolute best.

One study found that women who drank less wine had fewer cramps than those who drank more.

The endocrine system is simply powerful and elegantly complex. It's an organ system of glands, each of which secretes a type of hormone that regulates a particular function in your body—not just the hormones that give you cramps, make you bloat, or cause you to feel randy. Hormones affect your metabolism, the way your skin and nails look and feel, your ability to think clearly, how hungry you are, whether you'll have a period or a baby, your libido, and how much energy you have.

In order for your hormones to do their various crucial jobs, they have to work in harmony to achieve balance; but they can't get there if any of them are out of whack. So what makes hormones go haywire? FLO Blockers 3 and 4: our toxic environment and lifestyle (including too much stress and not enough sleep), and our modern diet (including processed foods, sugars, and caffeine). When even one hormone functions incorrectly, due to these factors, the imbalance creates a symptom, then another, then another. If they're not resolved, they can eventually create a chronic condition such as painful periods, endometriosis, fibroids, and so on. And if issues remain unaddressed for years, they can boost your chances of suffering from chronic inflammation-based conditions such as heart disease, diabetes, or infertility, depending on how well your diet and lifestyle have kept certain genetic factors at bay.

Your endocrine system is a series of glands that communicate with each other using hormones; think of it as a type of "chemical language." This is in fact your WomanCode in action! Not only do hormones tell all the systems of your body what to do—kidneys, liver, metabolism, digestion, nervous system, reproductive organs—they also have an impressive second job: self-regulation. When your body is inundated with endocrine disruptors that make its function more challenging, like being forced to digest processed foods or cope with burning the candle at both ends, your hormones try to find equilibrium so that your endocrine system won't break down.

In the short term, your body has checks and balances to compensate for too much or too little of any hormone; it's your system's *long-term* response that causes persistent symptoms and chronic conditions. As your hormones try to help your body get balanced again, they may instead overcompensate and create other imbalances. This will impact how much estrogen and testosterone, growth hormones, hunger hormones, stress hormones, fat-burning hormones, energy- and libido-related hormones, and sleep hormones it should be making to amend the situation. These extreme shifts in body chemistry aren't how your gorgeous system was meant to work. Unexpected swings cause its natural means of regulating hormones to break down. Eventually your endocrine system gets so confused that it no longer knows what balance looks like. It stops responding the way it should. That's when symptoms like heavy periods, fibroids, irritable bowel syndrome, insomnia, yeast infections, tender breasts, depression, weight gain, and others turn into full-blown chronic conditions like those you may be dealing with today.

Unexplained infertility represents the most frequent infertility diagnosis in women, encompassing up to 30 percent of all cases.

The Ultimate Partnership

You've seen her before. That woman who struts effortlessly down the sidewalk, practically gliding along the pavement. Her hair is shiny and her skin is flawless. She's got the perfect outfit—as if she stepped out of a fashion magazine—and she's adorned herself beautifully with Pinterest-worthy baubles. She's glowing and confident behind bright eyes, and she radiates energy with every move. Perhaps you work with this woman. She stands in her power and never hesitates to say what she thinks. She always goes after what she wants, and as a magnet for opportunity and making connections, she achieves whatever she sets out to accomplish. She speaks with clarity and wisdom; and when she talks, others listen.

You may think that this woman knows something you don't, or perhaps she hit the genetic jackpot. But you know what? This woman isn't any different from you. She wasn't born with any gift you didn't receive. She has exactly the same lady parts you do. The only difference: she's used them to create a life that's powerful, abundant, and radiant. She embodies that state I've talked about called FLO. Maybe you've experienced glimpses of FLO in your own life. Or perhaps you can't remember the last time you had one of those peak moments. Whatever direction you're approaching from, today my goal—the whole reason I wrote this book—is to take those moments and turn them into your daily experience.

This book is not about getting healthy for the sake of getting healthy. I say this because I've seen thousands of women go through my protocol over the past decade and heal from their conditions. So I know that if you picked up this book looking for a solution to problems in any of the big three categories (menstruation, fertility, or libido) and you follow the protocol, you will get better *and* keep future issues from popping up along the way. At this moment that may seem like all you could ask for. But I've learned over the years that there is so much more to life than attaining pristine health, and that ensuring long-term health requires choosing a bigger purpose. I want you to experience that for yourself.

Once you've understood the dietary and lifestyle changes that you'll be making (or have already begun to make), you'll see that WomanCode really is based on common sense: feed and move your body in ways that work with its natural rhythms. I want to help you tap into your personal best of physical, mental, and emotional health so that you can live the life you want to live, using your healthy body as a resource to create that life for yourself. A life where you're drawing in all of the good and radiating it back out so that you can share it with others. As a woman, living your personal best is your birthright, and I'm here to help you reclaim it. Here's how we'll do it:

- Identify your hormonal symptoms and help you see how issues you didn't suspect were hormonally related connect to malfunctions in your endocrine system
- Translate the language your endocrine system speaks—the language of hormones—so you can build a beautiful new relationship with your body
- Learn about the food and lifestyle habits that will help bring your endocrine system back into balance
- Reveal how connecting with your feminine energy and partnering with your body can help you create and achieve the life of your dreams

Once you get healthy, you'll start to realize just how the practice of planning your day and your life through the lens of what's best for your endocrine system allows you to be successful at getting more done with less stress and effort. This is what living in partnership with your body looks like. When you live in partnership with your body and operate with every tool that's naturally available to you, you experience your full potential. Your health becomes the platform upon which you can design a life with intention, passion, and purpose.

Take the Ovary Oath

So are you ready to do this? If you're going to start living the Woman-Code way, and get in your FLO, I'd like for you to vow on your soon-to-be-flourishing ovaries that you'll take responsibility for what you put in your body, home, and garden—and how you spend your time on Planet Earth. You're the only one who can keep your hormones safe, and it's a scary world out there. The U.S. Department of Agriculture says hormones in beef are safe, and yet research has repeatedly suggested that hormone residue influences infertility and breast cancer rates. The federal Toxic Substances Control Act hasn't been updated since 1976, and the current law is so weak that the Environmental Protection Agency (EPA) couldn't even use it to ban asbestos! (The law doesn't require chemicals to be registered or proven safe before they're put into use, and—legally speaking—it's harder to prove that a chemical's unsafe *after* it's been released than *before*.) Your boss makes you work over forty hours a week, and yet studies say women have more stress than men, due to juggling work *and* home duties. Big food brands swipe nutrients from your lunch and replace them with endocrine-disrupting chemicals such as genetically modified soy. There's a lot to be vigilant about.

....

The Ovary Oath

*I believe in aligning daily with my hormones and
using food as medicine to support them.*

*I believe in the power of my cycle and
hormones and know that they need to be cared for,
supported, and nurtured.*

*I promise to pay attention to the signals my body gives
me so that I can make small course corrections and
avoid larger breakdowns down the road.*

*I promise to use my body and health as a platform for
creating an extraordinary life in which I'm living my
purpose in the world.*

....

But we can't control what we can't control. What we *can* control is what we're eating and how we're living. By improving our cellular and physical environments with diet and lifestyle changes, we can impact the genes that cause the expression of conditions and diseases—and that's really exciting news, for you and for generations of women to come! So let's move on, now, to learning how to halt your avalanche of endocrine disruption once and for all.

One-on-One with Alisa

What do you feel is your biggest FLO Blocker in this very moment? If hormonal misinformation is your biggest challenge, then you are about to learn all about how the WomanCode inside of you is working on your behalf to keep you in the FLO. Or perhaps you feel that a long history of thinking negatively about your hormones and your body are to blame. If so, what messages have you inherited about your body and how it should look and act? Is your larger issue more the problem of food and lifestyle? Have you realized that the products in your home and the food you are eating are not allowing your WomanCode to perform optimally? Wherever you find yourself right now, the most important thing is to identify what those FLO Blockers are so you know where to direct your energy and attention in cleaning house! Rest assured that by the end of this journey into the world of your WomanCode, these FLO Blockers will be a thing of the past and will no longer prevent you from experiencing the gift of balanced hormones and a healthy body.

Success Story: Emily Whyte, 28

CONDITION: PCOS

I grew up an active, successful teenager who seemed to have it all. I was in impeccable shape, and to the outside observer my life looked perfect. I never had periods, and I was okay with that. In fact, I liked it. I wanted to have control over my body. I had way too many things to do to slow down and deal with menstruation. I wanted the power, the consistency, and the follow-through—with no messy emotions, no messy bleeding. Men had that. Why couldn't I?

It seemed to be so much easier to get around in the world without periods. So what if I had to take drugs for my acne and my unwanted hair growth? So what if I was continually anxious and exhausted? The drugs worked, and I kept up with my busy, important schedule. And on the outside it all looked pretty and perfect.

Then, at the age of seventeen, I was diagnosed with PCOS. One might think this would have begun the story of my healing, but it only took me further into the abyss of disconnection with my body. My doctors told me I had no choice but to go on the Pill. Phrases like "cancer danger" and "inability to have children" were repeated. The doctors promised that birth control wouldn't change who I was. They promised that this was the healthiest route—honestly, they said, the only way to treat my "disorder." For the next ten years I searched for doctor after doctor to find someone who might have an alternative method. They all fed me the same story: fear.

WomanCode burst into my life when I was at my wit's end. I'd actually been receiving their e-mail blasts for over a year without ever reading beyond the headlines! I just didn't believe that something so seemingly simple could have an impact. One day, I finally read Alisa's testimonial and something clicked. I began a six-month program, and for the first

Continued on page 52

time in my life I felt truly known. It wasn't easy to change my habits. It was terrifying to go off the Pill and have my doctor and family not really understand or support me. I even thought that giving up my "control methods" might somehow hurt me. But WomanCode gave me the knowledge and the support to begin trusting my own instincts again. Alisa and her team gave me permission to listen to something deeper. Now I've learned that control and power over the body are something very different from what a majority of the medical community teaches.

Today I'm finishing my ninth healthy and happy menstrual cycle in a row! And the truth is, every single aspect of my life has changed since I began my program. This is not an exaggeration. By taking the time to learn to listen and appreciate my menstrual cycle, I'm finding the deepest flow in my life, my career, my relationships, and—most importantly—my daily dealings with myself. Everything is easier. Everything is lighter. The energy I used to expend keeping it all looking so perfect is now flowing into enjoying my life.

And that, to me, is power.

CHAPTER 3

Girl Meets Body

In chapter 2 you saw for the first time that symptoms you may never have associated with your endocrine system before—such as migraines, acne, insomnia, weight gain, and constipation—can all be very much hormonally based. Still, this begs the question, How do you go from weekly sleepless nights or occasional breakouts to full-blown hormonal breakdown? As you'll see in a moment, when I explain how your endocrine system works, every organ and gland is intricately interconnected and works collaboratively with the others to produce every little life-sustaining function in your body.

The reason occasional symptoms have the opportunity to persist is that, due to lack of information, we're often unable to connect the dots between those symptoms and our hormones. (That's FLO Blocker 1.) So while issues such as cold hands, chronic respiratory infections, and eczema may seem like isolated symptoms to most people, they're actually telling you that your thyroid is underperforming, your adrenals are fatigued, and your liver isn't detoxifying the way it should. (These are all major parts of the endocrine system that you'll learn more about in a moment.) When there's a problem somewhere in your endocrine system, the other parts try to pick up the slack. Just as overworking a strained muscle at the gym puts that muscle and those around it at risk, the tendency for your endocrine system to overcompensate for problems weakens the system as a whole and makes you more vulnerable to hormonal dysfunction.

Another reason that symptoms persist is that we become desensitized to them. If you feel bloated or headachy after eating a meal and simply brush it off as an isolated incident, and do the same when it happens again, and yet again, you can quickly become so accustomed to feeling bloated that this sensation becomes your "normal." Over time you may notice these symptoms less and less. Even worse, you may lose the connection to the behavior that caused them in the first place (such as eating a food you may have an intolerance to, like wheat or dairy), and then of course you continue to engage in the offending behavior. When you're not able to read your endocrine system's messages, you can't effectively intervene, and quickly one symptom leads to another and then another until you're struggling with a much larger, impossible-to-ignore, and serious health issue.

If you're coming to this book with menstrual, fertility, or libido problems, the reality is that your mountain of symptoms has been piling up for years until they became a condition your doctor could diagnose. At the time you received a diagnosis, you may have felt as if a weight had been lifted: *Now that I know what's wrong with me, all I have to do is treat the symptoms to make it go away!* That's exactly how I felt hunched over medical journals when I ran my fingers across those four letters—PCOS—for the first time and knew in my gut that it wasn't all in my head.

Since then, however, you've undoubtedly fought an uphill battle. Since your diagnosis, you may have been throwing supplements, medications, special diets, birth control pills, and perhaps even surgery at the problem, trying to get it to disappear. I know you're frustrated, tired, and disheartened. That's because what you've really been doing is trying to address the problem at its surface instead of repairing it at its root cause.

When in sync, your endocrine system hums along in exquisite symphony. But when FLO Blockers—toxins in the environment, in our food, and in products we use, along with a stress-fueled lifestyle and a diet that deprives our bodies of essential nutrients—disrupt our endocrine system's natural opus, chaos ensues. A mismanaged endocrine system (the result of living out of sync with your body's innate wisdom because you never knew to do otherwise) allowed those symptoms to appear. Ignoring those symptoms caused them to pile up, resulting in a mountain of issues that have culminated in your current castaway condition. Shoveling them away with the prescription du jour hasn't done and won't do a darn thing except cause even more symptoms and despair.

I'm here to tell you that there's a much easier path you can take to descend into the valley of health, which is exactly what the Woman-Code method will help you do. With every meal, every day, you're going to address the issues that created the mountain in the first place. With every meal, every day, you're going to rebalance your endocrine system, which has been sending nothing but fuzzy signals and misfired messages. You're going to move the mountain altogether. The path is this: align with your hormones, allow your body to restore its own balance, and watch your symptoms clear up.

How I Fell in Love with My Endocrine System (and Yours)

Like many women with hormonal problems, I began my journey seeking help from countless practitioners with a variety of healing backgrounds and philosophies, ranging from the medical, to the complementary, to even the esoteric. And, as you know, nothing helped. Yet it really got me thinking: if my hormones weren't working for me, then I was going to learn everything about the endocrine system that I possibly could. At least then I would have a shot at understanding what was happening inside my body and why it had seemingly betrayed me.

As I educated myself about the endocrine system, I realized that it's not nearly as complicated and mysterious as its reputation. The endocrine system is our WomanCode, that's embedded in who we are and how we function. When you look at the various dictionary definitions of *code* there's no mistaking the link: "A system of signals . . . used to send messages." Your endocrine system is made up of a system of organs and glands that send messages to one another via hormones that determine how the system functions. Another definition: "A systematic collection of laws or regulations . . . governing behavior or activity." Your endocrine system functions in a completely regulated, predictable way and dictates every aspect of your behavior and physical and mental activity from your health, to your thoughts, to your mood, and so much more. The code inside your body makes you who you are. It's the most important code you'll ever understand because it's running the show of your life. And when you understand your WomanCode you gain access to deciding how, exactly, you'd like that show to go.

When I understood that there's a clear order to how the hormones operate when the endocrine system is working well, I came to see that I just needed to address each part of the system individually and in a specific order to get it functioning again. Until that point I'd been using a toss-the-spaghetti-at-the-wall approach—throwing a bunch of potential treatments at my symptoms and hoping something would eventually stick. But that's not how our

WomanCode works to allow the endocrine system to heal itself. All of the treatments I had tried were outside of my body, and yet I was looking for them to solve my problems. Instead, I had to understand that I needed to gain access to the code that was inside my body. It wasn't until I committed to learning the code, speaking the code, and working with the code that my body healed itself. When I started to put this program together for myself I asked: What does my body want to do? How does my body work? And what are the things I need to do in order to support its processes? In this journey, I deciphered the code and learned how my endocrine system works in order to get it working in the exact way it was designed to function. The endocrine system's methodicalness comes from the fact that the brain—the control center for your hormones—has to interpret so much hormonal information at one time that it needs to prioritize the importance of the various hormones in order to get anything accomplished. In other words, your brain is your endocrine system's ultimate project manager. Everything that happens in your body begins with a signal produced somewhere along your endocrine system.

When I started understanding the language of hormones, I experienced an enormous *Aha!* moment. (At that point I didn't know that it would one day be the basis for an entire career of helping other women heal their hormonal problems, too!) But finally, it made perfect sense to me why I had these issues and what I needed to do to improve them. The path forward was crystal clear, and it was a tremendous relief not to feel like a victim of my body any longer. My fear about my own body instantly melted away in light of the information and understanding I'd gained about my hormones. Instead of feeling like I had to wrestle my body into submission to get it to do what I wanted, I could step into partnership with my body. It was *I* who had been missing in action all along, not the other way around.

My new understanding gave me great hope that I would soon feel better; I no longer peered into a future where I would feel continuously worse.

I want *you* to feel this same sense of excitement I did, which is why I urge you not to skip over the science discussion just to get the dietary details. The education is just as crucial as anything else I can offer you. In fact, as you're reading this next section about your WomanCode, the inner workings of your endocrine system, I want you to feel inspired. I want you simultaneously to become more curious and to feel that all of your fears, weariness, and sense of victimhood and confusion about your body are being replaced by a sense of communion, partnership, and understanding. What's been crazy all along isn't your hormones, but the idea that you should be staying away from them—that somehow that part of your body is totally off-limits or that you need an MD after your name to understand them. What you're going to see, instead, is that once you gain the key to unlocking your WomanCode, the more you learn about your hormones and align your life with their natural patterns, the more incredible your life will become.

Once I understood the order in which the endocrine system functioned and the fact that there's a cast of characters (your endocrine glands) that influence your health to varying degrees, I realized that there's also an order in which things break down. The underlying causes of all hormonal problems work like a line of dominoes: when one part of your endocrine system is affected, the next collapses, and soon the one after that falls, and so on. They topple in exactly the same order of importance they follow when they're working well and when they're undergoing regeneration and realignment. To this end, here are the five underlying causes of hormonal problems in women, the way we break the integrity of our WomanCode:

Mismanaged blood sugar

Overexertion of the adrenal glands

Congestion throughout the pathways of elimination

A lifestyle that works against the patterns of your menstrual cycle

Separation from your feminine energy

The WomanCode protocol works in exactly the same order to bring about hormonal healing one step at a time to restore the natural intelligence of your WomanCode:

Stabilize your blood sugar

Nurture your adrenals

Support the organs of elimination

Cross-train your menstrual cycle

Engage your feminine energy

The fifth item—feminine energy—wasn't part of my original protocol. I added it about two years into my practice. I had started to witness that every woman who went through this process wasn't just getting healthier, she was also transforming every single area of her life. The question *Why?* stared at me in every single session. As with all things in my work, I was able to step back and take a holistic view of the endocrine system.

The first part of my research, when I was designing the protocol, looked at each individual moving part of the endocrine system—how each one worked, what they needed in order to do their job most effectively, and how they fit into a routine with all of the other parts. I then began observing the quality of the endocrine system as a whole and its effect on our behavior. From that broader perspective,

I saw that everyone's endocrine system creates an environment of constant change. In fact, I saw that my clients were making changes in *every* part of their lives as they became more attuned to the chemical changes happening within their own bodies.

When your endocrine system is compromised, you don't have good access to your innate nature of change. It's like a CD that's skipping—you can't move forward in other areas of your life when your hormones aren't moving fluidly. Now, think about the complexity of not having enough of certain hormones circulating in your brain, or too much of those hormones—you literally can't think straight. So how are you supposed to intelligently and strategically look at your life and create new ideas and connections when the brain doesn't have access to an ideal chemical environment? You can't!

But there's good news: I noticed in my clients and in my own life that healing hormonal dysfunction gives us the ability to tap into our power—the power of continuous change—a force that I came to

Learn to Love Your Lady Parts

From a WomanCode standpoint, "lady parts" are all of the physical structures that support the function of your reproductive system. These include the following:

- *Hypothalamus*
- *Pituitary gland*
- *Thyroid*
- *Liver*
- *Kidneys*
- *Pancreas*
- *Large intestine*
- *Lymphatic system*
- *Adrenals*
- *Ovaries*
- *Fallopian tubes*
- *Small intestines*
- *Uterus*
- *Vulva*
- *Vagina*
- *Clitoris*
- *Breasts*
- *Gallbladder*

identify as feminine energy. Accessing that power has since become the fifth and final step of my WomanCode protocol and is just as essential to your long-term health and healing as the other four steps. I've dedicated an entire chapter (chapter 9) to your feminine energy and how to engage it. I encourage you to come back to this idea time and time again as you live your life from a foundation of good health and begin to create change in every aspect of your life and the world around you.

From Your Head to Your Ovaries: Cracking the WomanCode

Think of aligning yourself with your endocrine system this way. When you're hungry, you know exactly what your body is trying to tell you. You don't feel your stomach growl or your energy sputter and wonder what's going on. No—you make a beeline for the closest source of fuel so you can satisfy your empty belly. In much the same way, you're going to be able to interpret your endocrine system's signals as seamlessly as you do hunger and give that system the TLC it needs to perform beautifully at all times.

The only way you can possibly get to know your endocrine system's signals as thoroughly as the physical cues you've been listening to your entire life is by gaining a much deeper understanding of how that system works. Once you've achieved that, it's easy to see how hormone misfires manifest as symptoms that vary wildly—from a foggy brain, to killer menstrual cramps, to chocolate cravings, and so much more.

All aspects of your endocrine system are involved in making or breaking how healthy you are in the category from which you're coming to this book: menstruation, fertility, or libido. What's happening in the five different endocrine support systems I'll break down in just a moment is the underlying reason why your period, fertility, or libido is failing you. This was one of the major discoveries I made when it came to treating my own gynecological issues. Instead of treating the symptoms, which was what every medical professional I consulted had been trying to do, I learned that if I worked with my endocrine system exactly as it worked, following its rhythm and supporting it with diet, exercise, and lifestyle habits, I could successfully restore it to normalcy.

I will help you do the same for your body. Keep in mind that the WomanCode protocol is not a quick fix; it's a lifestyle shift. What's so wonderful about the WomanCode approach is that once you resolve your symptoms with the protocol, the very same strategies you learn today will prevent your symptoms from recurring months or years from now *and* safeguard your body against new hormonal symptoms.

I'm sure you're already familiar with the term "mind-body connection," and perhaps you practice activities such as yoga, meditation, or biofeedback that strengthen this union. These practices are extremely valuable and have their roots in the original mind-body connection: your endocrine system. Hormones that flow from glands in your brain dictate what organs throughout your entire body—all the way down to your ovaries—do. The hormones that those glands release, in turn, govern every major process your body performs, from setting your internal thermostat, to metabolizing food, to keeping your heart beating, to regulating your mood, to determining your fertility, and so much more. So whether or not you ever find yourself in Downward-Facing Dog, nurturing *this* mind-body connection to improve its function is essential for living a healthier, richer, and more gratifying life.

Let's start at the very top of your endocrine system with your hypothalamus, an almond-size part of the brain that acts as your endocrine system's control center. The hypothalamus constantly receives information from your bloodstream about concentrations of various hormones. Depending on what it finds, it sends one of two hormones—releasing hormone or inhibiting hormone—to the pituitary gland, a garbanzo bean–size structure located just below the hypothalamus. The hypothalamus communicates *only* with the pituitary gland.

After interpreting the signal from the hypothalamus, the pituitary gland communicates with the remaining glands and organs of your endocrine system—thyroid, parathyroid, pancreas, adrenals, and ovaries—using a different hormone to converse with each. For instance, it sends out thyroid-stimulating hormone (TSH) to communicate with the thyroid, parathyroid hormone (PTH) to target the parathyroid, adrenocorticotropic hormone (ACTH) to speak with the adrenals, and follicle-stimulating hormone (FSH) and luteinizing hormone (LH) to signal to the ovaries. The target gland receives the pituitary's message and releases the hormone(s) it's responsible for producing.

Hormonal Buddy Systems

Those glands, organs, and hormones I listed above are the major players of your endocrine system, but none of them functions independently. There's a constant cascade of hormones flowing through your body at all times, and the different parts of your endocrine system are always working together to perform the countless functions they pull off every second of every day. So let's dive even deeper and take a look at how the parts of your endocrine system—especially those that matter most when it comes to the symptoms you're dealing with today—are supposed to function. I've learned that the best way to understand those parts, individually and together, is by looking at them as five different WomanCode zones. They are:

- *The blood sugar group*—pancreas and liver

- *The stress group*—hypothalamic-pituitary-adrenal (HPA) axis

- *The metabolic group*—thyroid and parathyroid

- *The elimination group*—liver and large intestine, lymphatic system and skin

- *The reproductive group*—hypothalamic-pituitary-ovarian (HPO) axis

WomanCode Zone 1: The Blood Sugar Group— PANCREAS AND LIVER

Unstable blood sugar is the most important underlying cause behind hormonal problems. The pancreas, liver, and brain function as blood sugar–stabilizing organs in the body. A full 98 percent of your pancreas (a six-inch-long organ tucked behind your stomach) is actually not an endocrine gland at all—it's an exocrine gland, which means it produces digestive enzymes to help your stomach break down macronutrients, such as carbohydrates and protein, in food. But that remaining 2 percent is a powerhouse. Its job: manufacturing the hormones that regulate your blood sugar levels.

When you eat refined carbohydrates (such as a candy bar or a bowl of pad thai), your body breaks down those carbs into simple sugars, primarily glucose. Your pancreas reacts to the abundance of glucose in your bloodstream by releasing the hormone insulin. Insulin's mission is to escort that glucose into your body's cells, which use the glucose to replicate their DNA, divide, and make new cells. Some glucose also ends up in your liver, where it's converted into glycogen, a form of energy your muscles rely on.

Your pancreas also responds to *low* blood sugar levels. When your blood sugar dips, which occurs when you don't eat enough or you wait too long between meals, your pancreas pumps out the hormone glucagon. This hormone tells the liver to convert stored glycogen back into glucose and releases that glucose into your bloodstream to bring blood sugar levels back up to par. This process makes sure that your brain, heart, and muscle tissues have adequate energy (in the form of that glucose) to do their jobs.

Although your body is programmed to restore glucose as a means of survival, you want to avoid putting it in a state of low blood sugar too often, especially if you're someone who's dealing with a variety of hormonal symptoms. As you'll learn when we look at the elimination group, your liver is responsible for breaking down estrogen that your body has already used and helping it leave your body. When estrogen lingers in your bloodstream, it piles up and throws off the balance your endocrine system is trying to maintain. This creates additional hormonal symptoms. Now, if the liver is frequently focused on converting glycogen into glucose because of low blood sugar, it's going to have less energy to spend on eliminating estrogen and other toxins. In other words, you want to use *food* to stabilize your blood sugar instead of relying on your liver to do it for you.

Controlling your blood sugar level is an extremely intricate and delicate seesaw that easily and frequently goes awry, which helps explain why nearly twenty-six million Americans suffer from diabetes today. Carefully selecting the foods you put into your body (the very premise behind my "every meal, every day" concept—more on that in chapter 4) is one of the best ways to keep your blood sugar levels as balanced as possible.

WomanCode Zone 2: The Stress Group— HYPOTHALAMIC-PITUITARY-ADRENAL (HPA) AXIS

The HPA axis is the switchboard for your body's response to stress. When stressed, your hypothalamus sends out releasing hormone, which stimulates your pituitary gland to secrete adrenocorticotropic hormone (ACTH). This surge in ACTH tells your adrenal glands (there's one located on top of each of your kidneys) to release a cascade of stress-related hormones, including cortisol and adrenaline. These compounds and the responses they trigger within your body evolved to help your cave-dwelling ancestors dodge dangers like saber-tooth tigers and encroaching tribes. Adrenaline, for instance, boosts your blood pressure and heart rate, while cortisol blasts glucose to your muscles so you have the energy to outrun lions and tigers and ward off loincloth-draped humans.

This fight-or-flight response was a lifesaving mechanism for your hairy predecessors back in the day. Today, however, your stressors—such as a hellish boss, a dwindling savings account, or a messy breakup—are unlikely to put your life on the line. Not recognizing that distinction, your HPA axis responds the same exact way it did ten thousand years ago, no matter the threat. When chronic stressors keep your HPA axis permanently on alert, that perpetual state of readiness can wreak havoc on your entire endocrine system and put you at risk of potentially deadly conditions such as heart disease and stroke. It can also cause insomnia, weight gain, fatigue, and challenge fertility and sex drive.

WomanCode Zone 3: The Metabolic Group— THYROID AND PARATHYROID

Your thyroid (a butterfly-shaped gland located at the base of your neck) is best known for determining your basal metabolic rate. What you may not know is that your basal metabolic rate is responsible for so much more than simply how many calories your body burns at rest. It also sets your heart rate, blood pressure, breathing rate, temperature, the speed at which your cells consume oxygen, and more. In infancy and childhood, the thyroid even supports bone growth as well as the development of the brain and nervous system.

Given the fact that your thyroid has a hand in so many elements of your health, you can see why it's so important to do what you can to take care of it. And yet one out of every two women will suffer a thyroid issue at some point in her life. One reason: your thyroid is incredibly sensitive to what's going on inside and outside your body, so even seemingly insignificant things like too few hours of shut-eye, too much chlorine in your water, or too many sugary caramel macchiatos can cause it to go haywire. But that's also the good news. Because your thyroid is so sensitive to what you put in your body and what you do with your body, you can easily support and maintain its health with simple diet and lifestyle changes.

The thyroid and parathyroid work as a team to monitor levels of calcium in your bones and bloodstream. The parathyroid churns out parathyroid hormone, which sweeps calcium out of your bones and into your blood. Your nerves and muscles (including your heart) rely on that calcium supply to function. However, left unchecked, the parathyroid may remove too much calcium from your bones, which can cause serious issues such as osteoporosis. As a safeguard, your thyroid produces the hormone calcitonin, which signals the parathyroid to redistribute some of the calcium it stole back into your skeleton. Maintaining the right levels of key micronutrients from food is essential for this zone's well-being.

WomanCode Zone 4: The Elimination Group— LIVER AND LARGE INTESTINE, LYMPHATIC SYSTEM, AND SKIN

Although these organs aren't producing hormones, they're essential for ushering hormones that have been circulating through your bloodstream out of your body. Can you imagine what would happen if the hormones your body naturally produced, as well as those found in the food you eat, medications you take, and products you use, *remained* in your body? Really, you would have an explosive hormonal experience if it weren't for your elimination group's ability to rid your body of these chemicals that, over time, become toxic to your health. (A buildup of estrogen, for instance, provides fuel for tumors to grow.)

Fortunately, the elimination group is your natural detoxifier. The liver breaks down hormones and other substances into smaller, more manageable molecules, which travel through your gallbladder and into your large intestine. There they bind with the fiber you consume in your diet and finally exit your body in the form of a bowel movement. In other words, when you go to the bathroom, not only are you disposing of the by-products of the foods you eat, you're also getting rid of chemical waste—broken-down hormones that otherwise would have overstayed their welcome and compromised your health.

The skin and lymphatic system have an excellent working relationship when it comes to getting cellular waste and hormonal overload out of your system quickly. Your skin is your largest organ and because of its concentration of pores provides a natural way for waste to leave the body—through sweat. Your lymphatic system is a superhighway for clearing away any cellular waste from your bloodstream, and the lymph node regions are where there's a concentration of action. This is why it's so important to keep the node areas flowing, as they are near key hormone-sensitive areas like breast tissue and ovaries. You most likely have already observed the effects of stress hormones leaving the body via the lymphatic system–skin partnership. Have you ever noticed a dramatic change in the scent of your armpit odor due to a stressful situation? This is your lymph–skin elimination channel trying to help compensate for dangerous levels of episodic stress hormones in the body. Without all of these ways for hormonal waste to leave the body, that delicate hormonal conversation would quickly break down as the hypothalamus would seek to suppress hormonal output.

WomanCode Zone 5: The Reproductive Group—
HYPOTHALAMIC-PITUITARY-OVARIAN (HPO) AXIS

Many women think of the menstrual cycle as something that happens solely below the waist, but the truth is, it's a sophisticated conversation that's constantly occurring between the ovaries and the hypothalamus and pituitary glands (both above the neck, another elegant example of the mind-body connection). The hypothalamus is constantly scanning your blood for levels of different hormones, including estrogen and progesterone, that your ovaries put out. Based on those concentrations, your hypothalamus tells the pituitary to send out two hormones associated with your cycle—follicle-stimulating hormone and luteinizing hormone—at just the right times and in just the right amounts.

While these hormones are directly involved in your fertility and your period, they also dictate how you feel on a daily basis—your mood, water retention, energy, and sex drive. The ratio of hormones at various points throughout your cycle sets up your emotional canvas—whether you'll be happy or cranky, energetic or lethargic today. In other words, to intimately know your cycle (which I will guide you through in chapter 5) is to intimately know yourself.

Tapping into the Signals of Your WomanCode

My goal in breaking down the various groups within your endocrine system is to help you gain a new appreciation for the complex processes your body performs each and every moment you're alive. With this newfound knowledge about your endocrine system, you may be wondering how you can start applying it to your own body and your own life. The most important thing you can do right now is become an observer of your hormonal health. Instead of dwelling on the big, annoying symptoms that you're experiencing—such as acne, low libido, or missed periods—trace those symptoms back to the five endocrine groups so that you can start noticing how well your endocrine system is performing and where it may not be working so well. At first this task may seem overwhelming, Please trust that you, as a woman, innately know how your body is supposed to be working. Your body is constantly in direct conversation with you, and nobody can tell you what's going on in your body better than you.

What does becoming an observer look like? Here's an example: You know that, ideally, you should wake up with energy and feel sleepy when it's time to go to bed. But if you have to tear yourself out from under the sheets (every *single* morning) and regularly experience a surge of energy when you're trying to fall asleep, these are clues that something—most likely in your stress group—is awry. If certain daily experiences aren't aligning with your expectations of how they should be going, write them down on a list that you keep in your purse or stored as notes in your smartphone. You can then use this list to better understand which of the five endocrine groups need your attention most (it's okay—and even expected—if the answer is more than one since they all work together). Gaining this familiarity with the different parts of your endocrine system and how each one is working is more helpful and empowering than focusing on your symptoms (as distressing and distracting as they may be). This exercise gives you the tools to better understand what's really going on behind the scenes. Furthermore, with this preparation, once you begin engaging the WomanCode protocol you'll be able to notice sooner and more seamlessly where improvements are occurring, based on how the experiences you've recorded change and improve.

My Promise to You

By now, you're already reframing your understanding of your own body. You can see how symptoms you used to dismiss as normal or simply annoying (even signs as subtle as dry skin and a languid libido) are actually hormonal. I want you to look back at the list of symptoms I asked you to circle in chapter 2 under the heading "Decode Your Lady-Specific Clues"—mental and physical symptoms, digestion and skin symptoms, and stress symptoms. Equipped with what you now know about the endocrine system, you can understand that these aren't inevitable "female problems" you're going to have to deal with for the rest of your life. They're indications that your endocrine system is out of balance—and now we're going to do something about it.

What's more, part of this beautiful process of understanding your unique biochemistry and aligning your diet and lifestyle with your endocrine system is discovering that hormones aren't just something your menopausal mom has to deal with. Hormones aren't only about hot flashes, sleepless nights, and mood swings. They're not even just about periods and pregnancy. There's a stream of hormones coursing through your body right now that's controlling everything from the rate at which your heart pumps, to how well your body assimilates nutrients from the meal you just ate, to your current mood, to how focused you'll be this afternoon, to how oily or dry your skin and hair may be . . . and so much more.

That's why it's so important to me to reach women who are in their twenties, thirties, and early forties (though peri- and post-menopausal readers, there's a great deal here that will help ease your transition, too). The sooner you step into this journey, partner with your endocrine system, and resolve your health issues with every meal, every day, the more magnificent your future will be.

SUCCESS STORY: *Kathryn Hiller, 35*

**CONDITION: Fertility Issues, Painful Periods,
Adrenal Fatigue**

When I started with WomanCode, I had painful periods, a hectic lifestyle, and irregular eating habits, and I was worried about my fertility. I knew that if I had some health coaching I could possibly see dramatic changes. On the plus side, I owned a successful Pilates studio in Fairfield County, Connecticut, had a wonderful husband of one and a half years, and was in great shape. I thought I had everything under control, and yet I couldn't conceive.

Soon after starting my WomanCode program, I discovered that my lack of self-care was making me a resentful, dehydrated, undernourished woman. Following WomanCode's simple recommendations, within six sessions I had developed a much better relationship with my body, and with my husband, simply because I was honoring myself. It was wonderful! When I actually slowed down to look at where my life was going, I realized that I deeply wanted a baby. Conception wasn't something we'd been able to accomplish before, but after going through the program, I was pregnant within a month! Now, at three months pregnant, I'm so grateful I didn't go the route of IVF.

What I've taken from this program is to honor my cycle, my own rhythm, and listen to my heart instead of my head. I know that without this program, I would not be pregnant now. I didn't know how to access the tools to reach this choice before WomanCode, and so I'm very grateful for this program. This baby is on its way because I made space for it. There was no room with my hectic, controlling life six months ago. I know that I will be a successful mother, wife, and business owner because I've been shown how to use the tools I already had. I feel like I'm in the flow of my life now.

This is a permanent lifestyle change that's easy to do and pleasurable to maintain, and it's never too late to start! Once you learn how to live according to the WomanCode plan, it quickly becomes second nature; when you feel good, you want to do everything you can to continue riding that wave of health, vitality, and openness to opportunities.

My promise to you, in the short term, is that you will feel more energized, experience fewer ad hoc hormonal fluctuations throughout the month, and kick weight and mood issues to the curb. Longer term, you'll protect and preserve your fertility and youth for as long as possible. And even more long term, everything in the Woman-Code diet and lifestyle protocol is designed to safeguard your health from the big four diseases—cancer, diabetes, heart disease, and Alzheimer's—down the road.

One-on-One with Alisa

There's no doubt about it: there's a ton of information packed into this chapter. An explanation of your entire endocrine system is a lot to digest. Please don't feel like you need to internalize it all at this moment. This is a book you can come back to multiple times throughout your life and always find new meaning and new relevance. Instead of feeling overwhelmed, focus on your curiosity and excitement about learning these incredible new things about your endocrine system. To help with that focus, answer each of these questions:

- What's one thing you learned about your endocrine system that you didn't know before?
- Which of the five WomanCode zones needs your attention most?

• What message is your body sending you through your hormonal conversation?

You may find that paying attention to your answers to these three questions is the best place for you to start. Trust that your body is guiding you to focus on what's most critical for you. Once you feel that you have a firm grasp on them, start over and identify another dimension of your endocrine system that speaks to you. With time and practice you'll come to understand and know your endocrine system in an intimate way so that you can partner with it to create improvement and change.

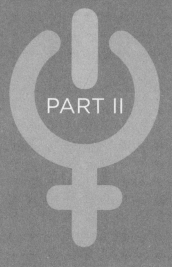

PART II

THE
WOMANCODE
PROTOCOL

CHAPTER 4

Access Your Healing Code

Most menstrual, fertility, or low-libido issues can be traced back to core dietary and lifestyle causes. This chapter will guide you through the first three steps of the WomanCode protocol—steps that directly address three of those underlying causes. You will learn to stabilize your blood sugar, nurture your adrenals, and support your organs of elimination. I'll explain how the systems involved support endocrine function, I'll help you take stock of how the systems are currently working for you, and I'll show you how to use food in ways that will support and optimize each of these systems' functions.

In chapter 3, you learned about your WomanCode as the form and function of your endocrine system. Now it's time to take our understanding of WomanCode one step further. If you think about your WomanCode like the combination to your gym locker, the correct combination always exists, just as your endocrine system is ever-present within your body. Whether you're able to access the contents of your locker depends on knowing the correct combination. In much the same way, these first three steps of the FLO-living protocol are like learning the combination to your endocrine system. Putting these three steps into action is how you engage with your endocrine system moment to moment and day to day. They're the steps you need to take, just like using the correct combination, to gain access to your WomanCode so you may support it for optimal health and vitality. After working with so many women over the years, I know each of us needs different levels of support and accountability when starting a program. As you go through this section, please remember you can join us on Facebook to share your daily experience of the reset at www.Facebook.com/FLOliving. You can also get more personal support for the WomanCode protocol through FLO Living's online hormonal improvement platform and virtual center. You can find more information about this in chapter 10.

Let's start with the basics. When your blood sugar, adrenals, and pathways of elimination aren't being cared for and nurtured with an "every meal, every day" approach, they quickly become unstable. The difficulty almost always begins with mismanaged blood sugar. Just as *low* blood sugar can compromise your liver function, so can *excess* glucose in your bloodstream. When you consume more sugar than your body needs, the excess gets stored in your fat cells, including those in your liver, which expand to accommodate the surplus. Excessive fatty deposits in the liver decrease the liver's ability to break down estrogen from your body, allowing that estrogen to hang around longer than it should.

Okay, now consider the fact that if your fat cells have expanded because of mismanaged blood sugar or chronic stress (excess cortisol from your adrenals will, over time, cause you to gain weight, too), you're going to have higher estrogen levels. That's in part because fat is hormonally active tissue and literally pumps estrogen into your body: the more fat cells you have, the higher your estrogen levels. With your liver doing a subpar job of sweeping estrogen out of your body and elevated estrogen levels thanks to an increase in fat cells, the stage is set for menstrual, fertility, and libido issues. In addition to disrupting your hormonal balance, estrogen drives many gynecological issues, both causing them and making existing problems worse.

Linking Your Symptoms with Your Endocrine System

Before we turn to the first three steps in the WomanCode protocol, let's take a closer look at why your body is experiencing the specific symptoms you're dealing with today and make some sense out of the quiz you took in the last chapter.

Why You Have Menstrual Problems

Genetics and nutritional factors determine how your body reacts to that mountain of estrogen. In my family, it manifested as PCOS. In yours, it may arise as fibroids, premenstrual dysphoric disorder, endometriosis, or something else entirely. It's fascinating to think that you were primed to develop your unique issue well before you were born or had your first period. For instance, my grandparents grew up in war-torn Italy and endured periods with little food. Epigenetically, this switched on the genes that made them, and now me, slow burners and good storers of glucose. Not only did I inherit the tendency to be a slow burner, I grew up consuming a typical Italian American diet of white bread, pasta, and cheese, which switched on the gene for me. In my grandparents' time, the slow-burning tendency helped them survive. Years later, though, in a time of abundance, it triggered problems for me. Unaware that my body was designed to handle only a small amount of sugar, I ate a carb-packed diet. This meant that for decades my blood sugar levels were all over the place, resulting in chronic internal stress, weight gain, and the backlog of estrogen I just described. Finally, the sky-high estrogen and hormonal confusion that developed as a consequence registered in my body as PCOS.

That's precisely why it's so crucial to do something about your endocrine issue *now*. (I will give you those tools later in this chapter.) Yes, you will feel better. Yes, you will have more energy. Yes, you will be able to get pregnant when you want to. But you will also, very likely, alter your epigenetic destiny so you can set your daughters and granddaughters up for easy, pain-free periods, meaning that they won't have to spend a single second suffering in your shoes.

Why You Have Fertility Trouble

In order to conceive, your body requires a very specific ratio of estrogen to progesterone. When estrogen levels become elevated by poor blood sugar control, adrenal fatigue, and congested pathways of elimination, the relative concentration of progesterone can become insufficient. When this ratio is disrupted, ovulation can become irregular as it does in perimenopause even if you're only in your twenties, thirties, or early forties. Also, without enough progesterone, your body cannot maintain a pregnancy; so even if you are able to get pregnant, inadequate progesterone levels will increase your risk of miscarriage. As any woman with fertility issues knows, it's not enough just to be able to *get* pregnant; you also want to set yourself up for a full-term healthy pregnancy. My protocol will enable you strike the optimal hormonal balance to do exactly that.

High estrogen levels impact your fertility in another, more indirect way. In the discussion above you learned how excess estrogen increases your chances of developing menstrual problems. Unfortunately, one major side effect of many of these problems is compromised fertility. For instance, PCOS prevents ovulation, which is of course essential for allowing an egg to be available to receive the sperm. With fibroids and endometriosis, there's a functional blockage within the uterus, which interferes with the successful implantation of an embryo.

That's why taking a pill to regulate your hormones when you suffer from menstrual issues isn't always a solution. Pills may temporarily (albeit chemically) regulate your cycle so you experience fewer symptoms. However, if your estrogen levels are not managed properly, those symptoms will always come back. Moreover, they will impede your chances of having a baby when you decide it's time. Additionally, women experience a sense of greater stress about these symptoms and obstacles to conception returning post-pill because they now feel that they have a shorter window within which to be balanced enough to conceive. The focus should be to view your fertility in the long term. Balancing your menstrual health immediately is the best way of preserving and protecting your fertility for the long term. The key is getting your blood sugar, stress responses, and pathways of elimination running smoothly so that estrogen can flow normally and you can experience abundant, flourishing, drug-free fertility.

Why You Have Low Libido

When you're exhausted because you've been riding blood sugar highs and lows, chasing deadlines or kids, or endlessly renewing the cycle of stress, getting busy with your honey is pretty much the last thing on your mind. At the end of the day you have just enough energy to eat more sugar (you can't help yourself!) and collapse on the couch. The equation is simple: low blood sugar plus chronic stress equals low energy and low desire.

From a physical standpoint, what your body has to do in the short term, when wading through the hypoglycemic and adrenaline-fueled aftermath, is so draining that it causes your body to do things that are not healthy. For instance, it tells you to eat more carbs even though you've already consumed too many (hence your hypogly-cemic state). As you consume those sugary carbs, your brain is working overtime to get the glucose it needs in any way it can and your body is slaving away, trying to flush reserved glucose out of your cells—and it's working even harder if you're a natural slow burner. All of this can lead to increases in cortisol levels. Long term, the excessive amount of cortisol produced from this vicious cycle has dampening effects on the production of DHEA, where the majority of your testosterone is derived, which is a key hormone in supporting your sex drive. Simply put, low blood sugar and stress

· ·

The Truth About Birth Control

Today, about twelve million U.S. women use oral contraception, commonly known as the Pill. For the right woman (someone without any hormonal disturbances), who's using it for the right reason (to prevent pregnancy), the Pill can be a wonderful thing. The problem is that so many women today use hormonal contraception for the **wrong** reason: to mask the symptoms of an underlying hormonal issue. According to a 2011 study by the Guttmacher Institute, based on U.S. government data from the National Survey of Family Growth, 58 percent of women use hormonal birth control for purposes other than preventing pregnancy. Of those:

- **31 percent use it to reduce menstrual cramps or pain**
- **28 percent use it to prevent migraines and other painful "side effects" of menstruation**
- **14 percent use it to treat acne**
- **4 percent use it to treat endometriosis**

The catch? Birth control doesn't actually cure any of these conditions. It simply alters hormone levels to diminish or eliminate the **symptoms;** the underlying hormonal problem persists. While on the Pill, you may very well are exhausting for your body; they leave little energy to spare for a satisfying sex life.

A low libido can be traced to numerous other causes, including limited knowledge about the biology of your sexual response and how to get the most out of it. The good news is that when you follow the first four steps of the protocol—address your blood sugar, adrenals, and organs of elimination, and live in sync with your cycle—your libido will improve dramatically. In chapter 8, I explain all of the necessary ingredients in revving your sex drive so that you can create the most sensual and pleasurable sexual experiences possible.

be able to go about your life without having any of these symptoms crop up again. However, if you decide to become pregnant and go off the Pill, you may find that getting pregnant isn't as easy as you thought it would be. That's because the underlying hormonal issue whose symptoms the Pill was prescribed to mask—an issue that may have been there for well over a decade, since you first went on the Pill—has never been addressed, and it's going to impede your ability to conceive.

The longer a hormonal problem exists, the more complicated it is to treat. So now, having gone off the Pill, not only do you have to direct your energy toward healing the issue, but it may take longer to do so than had you addressed the real problem originally. With women conceiving later in life today than ever before, this delay can pose a serious issue to your fertility, especially if you're in your mid to late thirties. You already had a narrowed window in which to conceive, and now you have the added challenge of healing a long-term hormonal issue that's complicated to resolve. With the right knowledge and tools it's doable—I help women through this problem all the time—but consider how much easier it would be now if you had known there was an underlying endocrine system disturbance to begin with and had addressed it when the symptoms first appeared, instead of covering it up with a daily pill for years on end.

Continued on page 84

One final thing to consider when it comes to the Pill is that there are millions of women walking around today with compromised endocrine systems who **don't even know it.** If you're one of them, those hormonal issues are even less likely to be identified if the Pill is silencing your symptoms. In other words, you could feel relatively healthy, go on the Pill for its intended purpose, and not realize that you have a serious condition that could block your fertility until you go off the Pill.

So my gripe isn't with the Pill specifically—it's with the fact that the Pill hides issues that you don't know you have or don't want to deal with. These issues will inevitably rear their heads sooner or later, especially when your fertility is on the line. If you're currently taking the Pill, for whatever reason, my advice to you is to work with your doctor to come off it for three to four months and observe what happens in your body. If your periods come back quickly, return each month like clockwork, and are relatively symptom-free, then it's your call whether going back on the Pill is the best decision for you. If, however, you go off the Pill and are plagued by heavy, painful periods, migraines, acne, fibroids, cysts, endometriosis, or other indications that something is profoundly off with your hormones, then you need to address your uterine and hormonal health **now,** especially if conception is in your future (within the next two to ten years).

It's also important to know that the Pill is not just between you and your uterus. It affects many organs in your body—ovaries, kidneys, liver, and heart. It impacts the quality of your blood. It changes your brain chemistry and alters the way your mind communicates with your body. It can have serious consequences for your physical health, moods, weight, libido, and personal relationships, and even your connection with yourself. In fact, a famous study—the sweaty T-shirt study—shows that birth control pills interfere with your ability to literally sniff out a mate who's an ideal genetic match for you. Previous research has found that the more genetically dissimilar two partners are, the lower their rates of miscarriage and the greater their chances are of having a healthy baby as well as happier relationships, more satisfying sex, and a greater likelihood of female orgasm. However, women on the Pill tend to (unconsciously) seek out men with more similar genes, presumably because *the Pill mimics pregnancy. As a result, if the body thinks you're pregnant, then you're not looking for a mate, you would already have one, and only be building friendships. In other words, the Pill hijacks your innate, hardwired ability to select an optimal partner. If someone you love was about to take a medication that did all that, you'd want to check in with her about it. So check in with yourself too—journal, talk with a friend, and investigate your body's response. Is the Pill right for you?*

The Pill has been an incredible gift to women of our generation and to our mothers. It has helped many more women have full participation in the workplace, choice and control in their family lives, and new adventures in sexual self-expression. It's been truly amazing. But the Pill is—as pills tend to be—a band-aid approach for women with serious hormonal imbalances. All women deserve to have healthy, powerful, and prosperous lives and to have the support they need to do so. Medication can only do so much and it's good we have more options!

*So, now, what's a girl to do? The first thing to do is to come to terms with your degree of hormonal sensitivity. If you're reading this book and struggling with any of these conditions, then the Pill may not be the best or even most effective treatment for you. The second step is to learn more about your own cycle. Understanding the hormonal dance your body performs every month is the key to choosing the birth control method that's best for you, and it's an amazing opportunity to practice prioritizing your own self-care. And because no system of birth control is foolproof (not even the Pill!), I recommend a combination approach: combine an intimate awareness of your cycle with any one (or two) of the array of barrier methods available. These methods provide effective protection without throwing your hormones into even more of an uproar. Finally, if you're not in a committed, monogamous relationship, whether you choose to be on the Pill, I can't stress it enough: always, always, **always** use a condom and dental dam. It's the only way to truly prevent contracting sexually transmitted diseases (STDs), which can impact your hormonal health and your fertility and even increase your risk for cancer.*

The WomanCode Protocol: Step 1—Stabilize Your Blood Sugar

We turn now to the heart of the WomanCode protocol: the five steps that will lead to improved health and life. Let's start with the most essential and easily disturbed underlying cause of your hormonal issues: your blood sugar levels. Stabilizing your blood sugar is the first step in my protocol.

What on earth does your blood sugar have to do with your gynecological situation? In a word: everything. As we've seen, your

WomanCode Recommended Methods of Birth Control

- **The male condom.** This has been around forever, popular because of its effectiveness at both preventing conception and protecting against STDs. The male condom is now available in a variety of colors and textures, as well as alternative materials for the latex-sensitive. Try Trojan or Avanti Superthin for a nonlatex option that feels just divine.

- **The female condom.** This is similar in function to the male condom, but designed to fit inside of a woman. Like the male condom, it's inserted just prior to penetration, and it helps to protect against STDs as well.

- **The Today sponge.** One of the most popular and effective birth control methods, it combines a barrier method (the actual sponge) with the extra insurance of a spermicide. Be aware that the sponge will not protect against STDs, so use it in combination with a condom. If you already know that you're sensitive to spermicides, this may not be the best option for you.

- **Diaphragm, cap, and shield.** Also barrier methods, these options—made of soft latex or silicone—are designed to fit snugly over the cervix. If you go this route, you'll need to visit your gynecologist for a fitting. One benefit: they're endocrine system performs all of its complex functions via the language of hormones. One of its main functions, first and foremost, is transporting glucose to your brain, muscles, and heart. If anything within *that* process is amok, you're going to have mismanaged blood sugar as the first problem; as a result, though, none of the other parts of your endocrine system will function according to plan either!

Now, consider this: not one client who has ever walked into my center has had well-managed blood sugar. Zero. The reality is that you cannot manage your blood sugar levels by accident. While sugar

reusable! (And so small and easy to carry . . .) Keep in mind, these babies are great for avoiding unintended pregnancies, but, like the sponge, they will not protect against STDs.

- *Vaginal contraceptive film.* This is one of the newest trends in spermicide. Similar to the ever-popular breath strips, contraceptive film is a thin, parchment-like sheet that dissolves instantly when inserted on or near the cervix. The film can be used alone or in combination with a condom, diaphragm, or sponge. The film is mess-free, as it doesn't produce any discharge. Each one-time-use film comes individually wrapped in a twelve-pack box. Film can be purchased over the counter at most drugstores.

- *What about an IUD?* For women who have already had children or are choosing a child-free lifestyle, then the Paraguard IUD can be a great solution, as it does not affect your hormonal levels. The Mirena IUD works differently, slowly releasing progestin, with the purpose of altering your hormone levels. For women who have not yet been pregnant, although more rare, there is a risk of infection or forming scar tissue in the uterus at the implantation site, which can make your successful conception more complicated. Again, the IUD does not prevent STDs and condoms make an excellent counterpart to this method of pregnancy prevention.

management doesn't require sophisticated testing or calculations (unless, of course, you're diabetic), if you haven't been consciously paying attention to your blood sugar and you've been eating typical American foods in typical American portions, or even the typically extreme health-conscious diet, your levels are probably out of whack. It's almost impossible to have healthy, well-controlled blood sugar without a little effort. (Soon you'll see that you're not off the hook if you haven't been eating *enough* either.)

As you learned earlier, your body breaks down carbs into glucose. Blood sugar management, as I define it, is monitoring and responding to your body's glucose levels, moment to moment, and taking the necessary steps to keep them on an even keel. This means carefully choosing what you put in your body from the second you roll out of bed until you power down your iPad at night. It also means knowing what to do if you've strayed from your ideal eating pattern, in order to bring things back into balance. In my case, for instance, if I eat a little too much brown rice, sweet potatoes, or pasta, I lace up my sneakers and head outside for a brisk walk around my neighborhood. Why? Glucose is energy. If I were to plop down on the couch instead, leaving my newly ingested glucose unused, my body would rush to churn out enough insulin to tuck that sugar into my liver and cells. But if I put my body to work, a good portion of the glucose in the meal I just ate is immediately used to power my muscles instead of hanging around waiting to be redirected. Exercise is a natural way of reducing the glucose load my body has to deal with so I won't experience severe spikes and drops after a carb-heavy meal.

Imagine a chart with a flat horizontal line—that's the ideal blood sugar stasis line. With mismanaged blood sugar, your glucose levels soar high above that line and then nosedive way below it—not just once, but again and again throughout your day. While it's practically impossible to ride that smooth line at all times (even eating an apple makes it jump slightly), with well-managed blood sugar, meaning you're feeding your body the right foods and at the right times, your levels gently undulate above and below the stasis line.

For those of you contemplating drastically cutting carbs or eliminating them altogether—don't. Glucose is your brain's primary source of fuel. Without it, you'll feel moody and lethargic and will even experience deficits in your ability to concentrate and retain new information. It's all about eating the right kinds and quantities of carbs in order to balance your blood sugar while feeding your brain. (Not to mention that eliminating or severely restricting complex carbohydrates increases the likelihood that you will have a hypoglycemic episode.)

Blood sugar management is truly at the heart of my "every meal, every day" approach. You can achieve beautifully stable blood sugar levels when you consciously and conscientiously select the foods you eat at every meal, every day. (I'll show you how.) But if you're choking down a veggie wrap sitting in traffic, or you forgo a meal altogether to finish a report, or you consume artificial sweeteners in diet foods and beverages, your blood sugar will immediately go haywire and you'll feel the effects for the rest of the day. Worse, the ripple effect won't end there. Since your entire endocrine system relies on your glucose levels hugging that stasis line as closely as possible, your body perceives mismanaged blood sugar as a stressor. This, in turn, sends your adrenals into overdrive and they begin to pump out a cocktail of cortisol and adrenaline—and the cascade of off-kilter hormones continues. And that's a snapshot of what happens behind the scenes following a *single* mindless meal. Repeat this daily, factor in your epigenetic response—the ways in which your habits trigger a hormonal response that results in particular symptoms based on your DNA—and it's easy to see how deeply interconnected what you eat is to how you look and feel and how your hormones perform.

Walking the Hypoglycemic High Wire

Most often, we talk about blood sugar in the context of elevated blood glucose levels, which can lead to insulin resistance and, eventually, diabetes. While this is a serious problem, it ignores a huge piece of the blood sugar management puzzle: hypoglycemia, or low blood sugar levels. This condition is just as detrimental to your body as its hyperglycemia counterpart on the other end of the spectrum.

Hypoglycemia is likely to occur through one of two quite different pathways. First, it may happen because you're on a perma-diet and consider coffee and a Luna bar to be a meal. If your body lacks adequate food intake, let alone sufficient carbs, your blood sugar levels will be chronically low.

The second way you're bound to be hypoglycemic is a little more intricate. It begins with overindulging in carbs. However, you don't have to polish off an Olive Garden–size trough of fettuccine alfredo to get too many carbs. Anything more than a modest serving—a scant half cup of macaroni, rice, or mashed potatoes—is enough to send your blood sugar soaring. (Check out a measuring cup. You'll be astonished at how little half a cup is.) In response, your pancreas pumps out a flood of insulin to bring your blood sugar back down by escorting that sugar—in the form of glucose—to the cells that are its end users. What often happens, though, is that your pancreas miscalculates the amount of insulin needed and releases too much; so instead of bringing your blood sugar to baseline, it gobbles up too much glucose and leaves you with extremely low blood sugar— despite the fact that you just stuffed yourself. This is where you get frustrated, berate yourself for having no willpower, and head to the pantry to refuel on peanut butter M&M's even though you ate a Chipotle burrito less than an hour ago.

But I'm going to let you in on a little secret: biologically speaking, there's no such thing as willpower. This is terribly important, because I see women beating themselves up all the time when they can't keep themselves from caving in to a craving. That negativity ends right here, right now. It's *not* about how much willpower you have. There's simply no way to win the blood sugar battle once you're already riding the hypoglycemic roller coaster; your hormones will win every single time. When you're in a hypoglycemic state, your brain—deprived of the glucose it needs—assumes you're in starvation mode. Your brain responds to the faux starvation by sending out ghrelin, also known as the hunger hormone, to get you interested in food. In other words, low blood sugar literally makes you hungry even if it's the result of overeating. Your body can't tell the difference.

Want to know something else that's disturbing? Some of us are more inclined than others to give in to temptation when our blood sugar levels are all over the place. A study in the *Journal of Clinical Investigation* compared people's brain responses to images of high-calorie grub. As expected, they found that when blood sugar levels dropped, everyone experienced a decrease in activity in the prefrontal cortex, the part of the brain responsible for controlling impulses. In other words, had the ice cream and hamburgers the volunteers were looking at actually been available, people would have been more likely to indulge when they were hypoglycemic. But the researchers noticed something else: once blood sugar returned to a healthy level in normal-weight people, activity in the prefrontal cortex kicked in and suppressed their desire for the junk food, yet this didn't occur in those who were overweight. They continued to crave those high-calorie foods anyway. This is why it's so crucial to smartly manage your carb intake: you may unknowingly be one of those who are more susceptible to cravings when your blood sugar is erratic. Keeping it stable with every meal, every day (whether you're overweight or not) will enable your pancreas to spit out only the amount of insulin required to move the glucose where it needs to go. This, in turn, prevents blood sugar highs and lows and therefore keeps everything from your mood to your cravings cruising on a sweet, even plane.

What Kind of Burner Are You?

Although the basic mechanics of how our bodies process glucose is essentially the same across the population, how efficiently we do this varies from one person to the next. Still, most people fall into one of two types: fast glucose burners and slow glucose burners. Fast burners' bodies are able to move glucose into their cells rapidly and then immediately grab that glucose when they need it for energy. Meanwhile, slow burners (like me) have compromised insulin receptor cells, meaning that glucose stays in their bloodstream much longer before making its way into their cells. Furthermore, once it finds a home, it requires much more energy to retrieve that glucose in such people than in someone who's a natural fast burner.

You're actually more familiar with this concept than you may think: when you're chatting with your friends about how fast or slow your metabolism is, you're actually referring to what type of burner you are—not what kind of metabolism you have. (Metabolism encompasses all of the chemical reactions that occur in your cells that help keep you alive.)

How can you tell what kind of burner you are? ID your type with this checklist below:

Fast Burners

- Tend to lose weight easily
- Feel anxious, dizzy, and headachy when hypoglycemic or hungry
- Overheat even with little exertion

Slow Burners

- Tend to gain weight easily and have a difficult time losing weight
- Feel irritable or foggy-headed when hypoglycemic or hungry
- Almost always feel cold—especially in the fingers and toes

Knowing which kind of burner you are will help determine how many complex carbs you can handle with your meals. Since glucose swirls around in a slow burner's bloodstream much longer, if you are a slow burner you require fewer complex carbs than a fast burner, who rapidly whisks the glucose into her cells and quickly becomes hypoglycemic if her carb intake is too low.

While you can't change the type of burner you are—a slow burner is never going to become a fast burner, and vice versa—you can improve your diet to support your body's ability to efficiently use glucose. This will make all the difference in everything from your energy levels to your hormonal balance to your overall health.

Taking Blood Sugar Management to Heart

There's one more reason why it's so crucial to get your blood sugar levels under control: because your life depends on it. By now you've heard that heart disease is the number-one killer of women. But did you know that more women die from heart disease than the next four causes of death *combined,* including all forms of cancer? And with more women walking around with out-of-control blood sugar levels than ever before, the risk continues to rise.

What's more, researchers are finding that women's hearts are more susceptible to damage due to sky-high blood sugar than men's are. In fact, one recent study found that women may face a *greater* risk for heart disease at *lower* blood sugar levels than men, meaning they're likely to develop blood sugar–related heart damage sooner, according to the *Journal of the American College of Cardiology.* And you don't have to be diagnosed with diabetes to be at risk: even when your blood sugar levels are elevated, but still below what's considered the threshold for diabetes, your risk of ticker trouble is equal to that of someone who already has the disease, the study found.

Scientists are still working to better understand the blood sugar / heart disease connection, but prevailing wisdom suggests that elevated blood sugar levels, over time, damage the blood vessels that carry blood to and from the heart. In addition, people with elevated blood sugar are more likely to develop high blood pressure and abnormal cholesterol levels and are more likely to be overweight than those with blood sugar levels in the healthy range, all of which also ups their cardiovascular risk.

SUCCESS STORY: Naomi Kent, 33

**CONDITION: Recurrent Urinary Tract Infections,
Adrenal Fatigue, and Anxiety**

I felt sick throughout most of my twenties and early thirties. I was always cold and exhausted, and I developed a urinary tract infection every three months or so. I was constantly on antibiotics but was never getting better, and none of my doctors could tell me what was wrong with me.

Finally, at thirty-one, I found FLO Living. Alisa asked me what I was eating and what my sleeping habits were like, and I came to realize that my lifestyle was responsible for my poor health. My high-sugar diet—I'd often have a bowl of Froot Loops after going for a run, and I frequently downed fruit juices and ate white pasta—were at the root of my unstable blood sugar levels and adrenal fatigue. I always thought that eating sugar would give me more energy, but it was my sugar levels yo-yoing all day that made me feel fatigued in the first place. On top of that, the sugar in my diet was feeding the bacteria responsible for my frequent infections. I remember sitting with Alisa and thinking that it all sounded so logical— how did I not know any of this?

I started seeing improvements in my energy and health within just a few weeks of starting the WomanCode protocol. What's more, I haven't had a UTI since 2010. I used to have problems sleeping, too. I'd lie in bed and my heart would be racing. I was constantly worried about everything and always felt anxious. These feelings stopped as soon as I started putting all the nutrition skills that Alisa taught me into action.

Naomi is a perfect example of how better health means better quality of life. Once you're feeding your endocrine system the foods it needs to functional optimally, you're free to channel all of your extra energy—as Naomi did—into living your life and having more fun at your job and with your friends.

Managing Your Blood Sugar All Day Long

Now you have the tools to understand, appreciate, and observe what your blood sugar is doing from one hour to the next. But that's not enough—I want you to have the tools to control your blood sugar so you can prevent hyperglycemia, hypoglycemia, and all of the symptoms (headaches, irritability, fatigue) that accompany both. Below is your blood sugar–stabilizing toolkit. Achieving stable blood sugar levels is an ongoing process that occurs throughout your day, and with these strategies, which easily become habits, you will feel great from morning to night.

Morning

- Upon waking, immediately drink at least 8 ounces of water. (If drinking room-temperature water on an empty stomach gives you a bellyache, try drinking hot water with a slice of lemon.)
- Eat breakfast within ninety minutes of waking.
- Don't consume caffeine of any kind before eating breakfast.
- Eat a protein-rich food with breakfast, such as eggs, a vegan protein shake, or smoked salmon.
- Minimize carbohydrates to 30 grams in the morning if you're a slow burner and no more than 50 grams if you're a fast burner. (A packet of plain instant granola contains 19 grams of carbs, ⅓ cup of granola contains 22 grams of carbs, and two slices of sprouted whole-grain bread contain 30 grams of carbs.)

Lunchtime

- Eat lunch within three and a half hours of breakfast.
- Consume the majority of your daily calories at lunch.

- Try to consume only one complex carbohydrate. For instance, have brown rice or black beans, but not both in the same meal.

- Incorporate at least one good-fat food, such as avocado, olive oil, or sunflower seeds. They keep blood sugar more stable and prevent you from craving simple carbs later in the day.

- Take a digestive enzyme (a form of nutritional supplement) so you absorb as much nutrition as possible from your meal. (I recommend Rainbow Light's Advanced Enzyme System.) If you notice a significant improvement in how you feel when you take a digestive enzyme, feel free to take it with every meal; but if you take it only once, make sure you take it with your largest meal, which should be lunch.

Midafternoon

- Eat a snack within two and a half to three and a half hours of lunch.

- Choose a nutrient-dense snack that will keep you satisfied until dinner. Some suggestions: rice crackers with avocado, hummus, or a slice of turkey breast; apple with natural peanut butter; goji berries and almonds.

Dinner

- Eat dinner within two and a half to three and a half hours of your snack.

- Create a meal that consists of vegetarian or animal protein and raw or cooked vegetables.

- Avoid grains and sugar of any other kind. If you consume sugar at night when you're least active, the resulting glucose is more likely to be stored as fat than used for energy.

- Schedule dinner so that you will be going to bed three and a half to four and a half hours after the meal. If you stay up longer, you're going to get hungry and will naturally crave sugary foods that provide quick sources of energy.

One-on-One with Alisa

Stabilizing your blood sugar starts with paying attention to your individual response to foods you're eating. After every meal, take a moment to ask yourself "How do I feel?" It sounds simple, but be sure to push yourself for a descriptive, physical, and embodied answer—it doesn't need to be more than a word. Do you feel good? Tired? Gassy? Bloated? Energized? Full? This is the beginning of a life-long daily inquiry you'll be practicing in the FLO. When you start to ask it at every meal, every day it becomes your second nature. And when you know how different foods make your body feel, it will become easier to choose those that keep you feeling well because you've experienced and noticed their effects in your body. Similarly, it will become easier to avoid those that produce negative results because you will have consciously identified what those are and you won't want them anywhere near your improving health. Remember to ask yourself the question after beverages, too!

The WomanCode Protocol: Step 2—Nurture Your Adrenals

I mentioned earlier that your adrenal glands perceive mismanaged blood sugar as a stressor. Following the rules above to get your blood sugar under control will take you a huge leap toward balancing your adrenals—you'll be wiping out a major factor that's currently making it impossible for them to function normally.

But I'm pretty certain that off-the-charts blood sugar isn't the only stressor in your life. If you're like most modern women living in the twenty-first century, juggling a fabulous bag filled with iGadgets that keep you connected to all your obligations, you're probably under a barrage of stress from a slew of different sources. Keep in mind that whether those stressors are life-threatening or not (and chances are that few, if any, are), your adrenals react with the same hormonal response, meaning they're permanently on orange alert. But your adrenals were designed to endure the occasional stressful outrun-a-tiger sprint—not the marathon of chronic stress most of us are running. Unfortunately, spending months, years, and decades living in this hair-trigger state sets you up for a condition known as adrenal fatigue.

In its early stages, adrenal fatigue is characterized by ongoing tiredness and a general lack of vitality. Other telltale signs include acne, weight gain, insomnia, depression, increased susceptibility to colds and other infections, and sugar cravings. For many women, adrenal fatigue has become such an everyday experience—their new "normal"—that they don't even realize they could correct this and feel better.

When I think about the most severe stage of adrenal fatigue, one woman, a CEO of a health company, comes to mind. Her adrenals were so fried from years of chronic stress that she used to wake up in the morning with heart palpitations and a cold sweat. That's because the normal surge in cortisol that naturally lulls us out of sleep was traumatic for her body. Even though she knew, rationally, that she wasn't in any kind of danger, her body couldn't tell the difference. Her adrenals had become so hyper-responsive to every type of stressor that even the simple act of waking up in the morning triggered a full-blown panic attack. Then she'd have to drag herself through most of the day, pumping herself full of coffee and Diet Coke just to be able to function at a quasi-normal level. Her libido was nonexistent and she lived in a perpetual state of anxiety.

Whether her symptoms resonate with you or you simply want more energy to get the most out of life, your adrenals are the place to start. When your adrenals are functioning optimally, you wake up feeling energetic and optimistic. You seek out opportunities to engage your mind and your body because you have the vigor to do more, to create more, and to be more.

Peeling Back the Adrenal's Layers

Although we most commonly associate the adrenals with stress, they have a variety of other important functions in the body. To better understand all that your adrenals do, it's helpful to know the roles that the two parts of your adrenal glands—the adrenal cortex (the outer layer) and the adrenal medulla (the inner layer)—play.

The Adrenal Cortex

Remember the hypothalamic-pituitary-adrenal (HPA) axis that I described in chapter 3? Well, it comes into play again here. The cortex doesn't function of its own accord; rather, the hypothalamus signals the pituitary gland to secrete hormones (the important one, in this context, being adrenocorticotropic hormone, or ACTH) that control the adrenal cortex's output.

The cortex itself is further broken down into three microscopic layers or zones. Based on the unique enzymes located in each of these zones, they secrete different hormones that have various effects in the body. They are:

- *Zona glomerulosa.* This outermost layer produces the hormone aldosterone, which helps regulate your blood pressure and protects the sodium/potassium balance within each of your cells—a balance that allows cells to survive, divide, and remain intact. You can't survive without this hormone.

- *Zona fasciculata.* This middle layer churns out cortisol. Your body relies on a certain amount of cortisol coursing through your bloodstream in order to maintain your circadian rhythms (more on that in a moment) and mobilize stored fats, proteins, and carbohydrates from your cells when you need them for fuel.

- *Zona reticularis.* This innermost layer produces dehydroepi-androsterone (DHEA), a precursor to androgens—estrogen and testosterone—in men and women. In women, 90 percent of our testosterone is manufactured from DHEA in this part of the adrenals. This hormone is crucial in both men and women for maintaining and building fat-frying muscle mass, boosting your libido, supporting your energy, protecting your skeleton, and safeguarding your mental health and cognitive function as you age.

The Adrenal Medulla

The inner layer of the adrenal gland is the control center for your fight-or-flight response. The hormones it puts out set off your body's physical response to stress. When stressed, the adrenal medulla sends norepinephrine into your bloodstream, which restricts your blood vessels and increases your blood pressure. Meanwhile, epinephrine (a.k.a. adrenaline) boosts your heart rate

How to Exercise with Adrenal Fatigue

If you have recurrent adrenal fatigue, you probably have a particularly complicated relationship with exercise. Due to high levels of cortisol and chronically unstable blood sugar levels, you may be carrying some extra weight. So, of course, you want to exercise to help shed that weight. However, pushing yourself too hard in the gym when you're already struggling with exhaustion can cause even more stress and thus leave you feeling even more depleted. The solution may seem counterintuitive, but it's very much aligned with the endocrine system: exercise more gently and for shorter periods of time.

Here are my specific exercise recommendations when you're working to heal adrenal fatigue:

- *Three days a week do brisk walking/jogging intervals for a total of twenty minutes. Walk briskly for two minutes; then jog for thirty seconds. That's one interval. Do eight total.*

- *Two nonconsecutive days per week do a full-body strength-training work-out with weights for twenty minutes. Choose exercise pairings that combine multiple muscle groups, such as squats with overhead presses, lunges with bicep curls, side lunges with lateral raises, pushups and crunches. Do two sets of twelve reps for each exercise. Start with five-pound weights and work up to about ten pounds.*

- *Rest two days per week, which can include gentle yoga or walking when feeling better.*

Why this works: the cardio component (the walk/jog intervals) is long enough and intense enough to help you burn fat, but without causing the and directs blood flow away from your organs and toward your muscles, the purpose being to enable you to outrun a teeth-baring Rottweiler.

adrenals to become overstimulated. When you're recovering from adrenal fatigue, anything longer than twenty minutes causes cortisol levels to rise, so be vigilant about stopping your exercise at that mark even if you're used to pushing yourself harder or longer. The strength-training component will help increase lean muscle mass, which aids blood sugar stability because your muscles consume glucose for fuel; in turn, this "legitimate" use of glucose will take the strain off your adrenals because your bloodstream will no longer be bombarded by glucose. Combining several muscle groups with each exercise allows you to fit a total-body workout within that twenty-minute limit to maximize your time.

You'll know this workout is working for you when you feel energized instead of drained after you exercise. Never work out on a completely empty stomach; have something small such as an almond yogurt or green juice beforehand. Try to schedule your workouts for first thing in the morning or midday. Since women with adrenal fatigue tend to have inappropriate cortisol spikes—these occur when you're trying to fall asleep instead of first thing in the morning, as they should—morning workouts will, over time, fix this problem. In fact, waking up with energy will be the sign that your adrenals are well on their way toward healing. At that point you can increase the time or intensity of your cardio and strength-training workouts. If you wake up in the morning without an alarm clock and feel like getting up and moving, it's time to work up to thirty, forty-five, and eventually sixty minutes of cardio, and to adjust your strength-training workout by increasing the amount of weight you're lifting and upping the duration to thirty minutes per session. Even when your adrenals are healing, continue to take those two rest days each week. When you're feeling well, do some gentle yoga or take a leisurely twenty-minute stroll on those days.

Making the Circadian Connection

Every gland in your body maintains its own circadian rhythm through-out the day. By that I mean there are times when they're more active and times when they're at rest. This is what the science of chronobi-ology addresses. While most of these rhythms are barely noticeable, it's impossible to ignore when your adrenals are off. When they're functioning normally, the adrenal glands are most active between 8 A.M. and 8 P.M., with a big surge to wake you up in the morning and another key surge midday. It's no surprise why they evolved this way: your adrenal glands are in sync with the sun so that you have the most energy during daylight and wind down when the sun sets.

However, with chronic stress, you're often asking your adrenals to secrete cortisol during parts of the day when it would normally be dropping off. Your body adapts and, over time, your cortisol surges come later and later. One of the very first indications that a client has adrenal fatigue is when she tells me that she's become a night owl and can't fall asleep without popping Ambien tablets like Tic Tacs. Do you remember the CEO with severe adrenal fatigue that I mentioned earlier? She got most of her work done in the hours after 10 P.M.—her adrenals were so out of sync with what was normal that, after being a zombie all day, she perked up when her cortisol finally kicked in right when she was supposed to be going to sleep.

Soothing Stress Naturally

There are two kinds of stressors: internal and external. Internal stress-ors are those that disrupt your body's normal, healthy patterns and prevent you from accessing your WomanCode benefits—things such as mismanaged blood sugar, inadequate sleep, lack of physical activ-ity, and even the absence of orgasms. External stressors are those that occur outside of your body but have a real physiological and psychological impact on your well-being. In the chart below, I've outlined some of the most common internal and external stressors with action plans on how to minimize the toll they take on your body's stress response and your overall health.

Stress R$_x$

Internal Stressors	Adrenal R$_x$
Hypoglycemia	Plan the day with food in mind. Don't go more than three and a half hours without eating. Never leave home without emergency snack packs such as dried fruit and nuts, gluten-free granola bars, or pieces of fresh fruit such as apple.
Irregular sleeping patterns	Download a sleep app like Lark. Buy an alarm that gradually lulls you out of sleep with light (instead of jarring you awake with sound). If you have trouble falling asleep, try taking an herbal product such as chamomile or passionflower two hours before bed—they exert a relaxing effect on the HPA axis to help calm your mind and body.
Physical inactivity/ muscle tightness	Don't leave all your activity for when you're at the gym—find opportunities to move throughout your day. For instance, take periodic breaks to stretch at your desk: stand up, reach your hands to the sky, then touch your toes; repeat several times. Stand and twist your torso side to side. After lunch take a walk around your office or, if possible, head outside for a brisk walk even if it's only for five minutes. Download a yoga app.
Lack of regular orgasms	Orgasms provide a huge cortisol flush for the body to help relieve stress. Make time during the week to regularly self-pleasure. Avoid the temptation to use toys—it skips a crucial stress-relieving step called tumescence, where the tissues become engorged with blood. For tips on how to manually self-pleasure, check out the book Getting Off by Jamye Waxman. For women with lagging libido, try Zestra, an herb-based gel that you apply to the clitoris. Within thirty minutes, blood flow increases, which boosts desire as well as the ability to climax.

External Stressors	Adrenal R$_x$
Opening bills	Create a pleasurable ritual: for example, light a candle and put on music that you enjoy. Take steps to become a better money manager. Visit a website designed to help women take control of their finances with budgets, financial goal-setting, investing information, and access to experts who can help you further.
Commuting	Get your om on: download meditation tracks on iTunes. Make any experience more pleasurable while you have to endure it—download books or create playlists of music that you enjoy. Studies find that anticipating and listening to music that you love causes the brain to release the feel-good hormone dopamine, which makes you feel less stressed.
Coping with a difficult relative	Before spending time with a stress-inducing person, set the intention to not take anything he or she says personally. If you always leave an encounter feeling angry or hurt, begin to set boundaries with that individual. (For strategies on how to create boundaries, see chapter 9.)

One-on-One with Alisa

With some simple planning you can feel like you're in charge of your stress instead of your stress controlling you. In the stressor chart above I've offered some useful tools to help you get started. Now the power is in your hands. Look at the chart again. Pick the one internal and one external stressor you're most likely to encounter in an average week. Then select one suggestion for each of those stressors and try putting them into action for one week. If a particular strategy is a good fit for you, continue using it as needed. If you feel that another strategy might be more appropriate for you, start experimenting with that one, too. This is an ongoing project of learning how you can best cope with the stressors that occur in your life in order to minimize the impact they have on your endocrine function. Get creative: if you come up with other ways to deal with stressors, by all means make them your go-to responses. The key is to stop the cycle of stress by looking for opportunities to calm your nervous system and protect your endocrine system against the damage stress can create.

The WomanCode Protocol: Step 3—Support Your Organs of Elimination

The legend goes that at one time the most important person in the ancient Chinese emperor's court was the royal physician, who had the very critical task of inspecting the emperor's morning bowel movement. This Chinese medical doctor's role was dedicated to creating the emperor's daily meal plan and itinerary of activities based on his daily inspection. As potentially unpleasant as that may sound, and regardless of the legend being true, the physician would have been working in accordance with the very practical tenants of Traditional Chinese Medicine—that we can observe so much about our health from our own bodies. Our stool is an important indicator of our overall health. What's more, it's one of the only things we can actually *examine* to determine where our health is headed. Whereas you're unlikely to know whether something is off with your blood sugar and adrenal output until a problem manifests into physical, mental, and emotional symptoms, the signs of congested elimination are literally in front of your eyes every single day (as long as you don't flush first!).

When clients first come to FLO Living, I ask them to fill out an intake form so I can learn more about them and what they're going through. One of the questions asks, "What are some additional symptoms you experience that are unrelated to your menstrual/fertility/energy or libido problems?" In this space, many women jot down things such as eczema, irritable bowel syndrome, acne, constipation, diarrhea, or rosacea. It's not a trick question, but it highlights a simple reality: many people don't think of GI or skin issues as being hormonally related.

But they are.

When your pathways of elimination are congested, your body cannot get rid of toxins (such as the endocrine-disrupting FLO Blockers I mentioned in chapter 2) as well as the natural buildup of hormonal by-products that occur with normal metabolism. Now pile on the issues of mismanaged blood sugar and adrenal fatigue, which further interfere with your body's ability to Swiffer its own system, and you've got an open invitation for hormonal imbalance.

The Four Pathways of Elimination

Your stool isn't the only way your body gets rid of toxins. In fact, there are four distinct, though interconnected, pathways of elimination. What follows is a look at each one (with the liver and large intestine addressed together) and how you can tell whether they're working optimally or not.

Liver and Large Intestine

Consider the liver and large intestine your internal garbage processors, compacting and moving the big stuff such as digested food, toxins, chemicals, and hormonal waste every single day. Chances are you never gave much thought to your liver before, but after what I'm about to explain, there's no doubt you'll start thinking about that organ in a whole new way and seeking ways to support it every way you can, every single day.

The liver's primary purpose is to convert fat-soluble toxins (most toxins *are* fat-soluble) into water-soluble waste through a two-step process so that your body can excrete them via sweat, urine, and bowel movements. Toxins include chemicals in your diet and environment, such as pesticides, insecticides, dry-cleaning chemicals, alcohol, cosmetics, and household cleaning products, as well as hormonal waste—that is, hormones your body has already used and needs to get rid of. Hormones are fat-soluble because that allows them to stay in the body longer; if they were water-soluble, you'd eliminate them all the time and they'd never have a chance to carry out their job. The liver is responsible for moving hormones along once they've fulfilled their duty.

In the first phase of detoxification, the liver breaks down fat-soluble toxins into multiple components using nutrients such as glutathione, B vitamins, and C vitamins—nutrients stored in the liver from the foods that you eat. These multiple components, called free radicals, become more toxic as a whole than the original toxin the liver broke down in the first place. Due to this toxicity, it's essential that the second phase of detoxification kick in as quickly as possible; the goal is to minimize the damage these free radicals could do if they stuck around too long. In the second phase, selenium and amino acids in the liver (also stored from your diet) combine with these free radicals to make them harmless and water-soluble.

Ideally, once your liver transforms a toxin from a fat-soluble to a water-soluble molecule, it enters the gallbladder, mixes with bile, and leaves the body via the large intestine. The last thing required to complete this journey is an adequate source of dietary fiber in the large intestine to bind with the waste to make sure it leaves quickly.

Given the liver's two phases of detoxification and the necessity of ample fiber to properly eliminate toxins from your body through the large intestine, you can see just how critical it is to have adequate dietary intake of these micronutrients. Studies have found that you can't simply supplement with glutathione, vitamin B, vitamin C, amino acids, or selenium and expect the organs of elimination to function optimally. These nutrients don't readily become bioavailable when you take them as supplements; if you eat them as they naturally occur in foods, the body can more easily recognize them. Not only is it important to consume enough just so these organs work in the ways that they should; it's also critical to support both phases of detoxification, because if you're lacking in the nutrients required for phase 2 you risk exposing yourself to a greater degree to the toxins that your liver helped create in phase 1.

The last place you see this process being successful, the final phase, is when you wake up in the morning, have a glass of water, and feel the urge to have a bowel movement within about twenty minutes of waking. If it's longer than that or if you require a cup of coffee in order to go to the bathroom, then you're constipated (yes, even if you eventually go later that day). The reason is another example of chronobiology inaction: your liver goes into self-cleaning mode from 3 P.M. to 3 A.M. Your first bowel movement should happen soon after waking, because the liver has been working for the past twelve hours to get rid of yesterday's waste. Many people don't realize that constipation is more than a simple annoyance. The lining of your large intestine is osmotic in nature, meaning that things can travel in and out through the membrane. If you don't have an efficient transit time because your liver or large intestine is congested or you're lacking the necessary nutrients for them to perform their functions efficiently, the toxins and other chemicals working their way through this pathway can become reabsorbed into your bloodstream and continue circulating throughout your body. It's essential that *all* toxins and hormones be removed, and quickly. In particular, if you're not metabolizing, breaking down, and removing estrogen as efficiently as possible, an excessive amount will accumulate in the bloodstream and lead to menstrual, fertility, and libido issues.

	For the Liver	For the Large Intestine
Elimination Rx	*Fill your diet with foods that naturally aid the liver's detoxifying processes. These include good-quality protein (supplement with amino acids if you're a vegan), glutathione (found in carrots, broccoli, avocado, spinach, apples, asparagus, and melon), selenium (found in oats, Brazil nuts, poultry, eggs), and plenty of cilantro (which contains linalool, a compound that works to cleanse the liver)—add it to smoothies, salads, and other dishes for powerful liver detoxification.*	*Be sure to consume plenty of soluble fiber, found in oat bran, barley, nuts, seeds, beans, lentils, and peas. It works like an internal Swiffer to clear out your large intestine.* *Inspect your bowel movements. Ideally, they should be medium brown in color, curved, and smooth. In standard toilets, they should float briefly.* *Avoid treatments such as colonics. They're disruptive to your intestinal flora and are a short-term quick fix that can mask symptoms indicating an underlying hormonal issue that needs to be addressed. They're also potentially dangerous and can rupture the lining of your intestine.*

Skin

Your skin is your body's largest organ, so it's also, naturally, the largest organ of elimination. It has to handle whatever the large intestine and liver are unable to eliminate. It does so by excreting waste, to the best of its abilities, via sweat.

Have you ever noticed that when you feel stressed or upset, the sweat from your armpits smells especially foul? That's a surefire sign that your pathways of elimination are congested and your skin is trying to dispel the toxins that your other organs couldn't handle. Your skin is the *last* place symptoms show up when you're experiencing elimination issues. If you develop cystic acne, rosacea, or eczema, it's often a sign that the other systems haven't been working well. I encourage you, as much as possible, to avoid topical creams and other treatments (most of which only complicate the problem anyway) for these skin issues and instead follow my four-day cleanse (starting on page 126), which will help decongest the liver and large intestine. Watching your skin clear up is one of the most obvious ways of understanding just how much control you have over making sure your pathways of elimination are open and clear.

	For the Skin
Elimination R$_x$	*Occasional trips to steam rooms, saunas, and cedar baths can be extremely cleansing for the skin. (Avoid these if you're pregnant, trying to become pregnant, or have high or low blood pressure.)*
	When taking a shower, alternate the temperature from warm to very cold a few times. This causes skin cells to expand and contract, forcing fluid and toxins out of the skin.
	Exfoliate with a hot washcloth or sea-salt scrub a few times per week. This removes the layers of dead skin cells that prevent pores from releasing toxic waste from the skin.

Lymphatic System

The lymphatic system is a network of organs, nodes, ducts, and vessels that produce and transport lymph, a fluid made up of white blood cells. This network is a major component of your immune system. You may not automatically associate the lymphatic system with elimination as you would the liver or the skin, but it plays a huge role in detoxing the body. The lymphatic system sweeps up metabolic waste, toxins, dead cells, and excess fluid from your organs and deposits them into your bloodstream, which eventually transfers them to the liver and large intestine. But if your lymphatic system becomes clogged, the organs and parts of your body that normally deposit their waste into it become backed up and blocked, too.

When working efficiently, your lymphatic system directs white blood cells to germs and other invaders and helps you fight off infections. But when it's congested, the lymphatic system has the opposite effect: the fluid attracts these same viruses and bacteria and transports them throughout your body, dumping them into your bloodstream, and putting you at even greater risk of infection. People with lymphatic congestion issues are also likely to experience inflammation-related conditions such as allergies, high blood pressure, and chronic sinusitis, and they can develop autoimmune conditions such as rheumatoid arthritis and lupus.

	For the Lymphatic System
Elimination R$_x$	*Consider keeping a small trampoline (also called a rebounder) in your home and/or office and use it a few minutes at a time several times per day. It provides a gentle massage of lymph through the lymphatic system so that the fluid can be pushed out through your lymph nodes.*
	Keep crucial lymph-node-dense areas, such as the armpit and groin, clear of toxins. Make sure all products you use, including sanitary pads, are unscented. Avoid antiperspirant. Wear underwear that has a cotton liner, not synthetic. Minimize use of shapewear—wear it only occasionally for short periods of time, as it may block the flow of fluids trying to leave your body.

Four Days to Reset Your Woman Code

Now that you've learned about the first three phases of the FLO protocol, have addressed blood sugar stability, and have been work-ing on minimizing stressors, it would be excellent to take on this gentle food-based cleanse to help reset your pathways of elimina-tion, stabilize your blood sugar, minimize internal stress, and recali-brate your endocrine system for optimal performance.

A Weighty Matter

If you're like many women with endocrine fallout, it may seem like your body is hanging on to an additional five, ten, or even twenty pounds for dear life. No matter how little you eat and how much you move, those excess pounds refuse to budge. Sound familiar? Well, you may be relieved to learn that there's a physiological reason for this—and you'll be even more relieved to find out that there's a solution for it, too. (And it doesn't involve a crazy deprivation diet or super-intense boot-camp workout either!)

The root of the problem lies in your liver. As we have seen, the liver is responsible for removing toxins from your body, and it does this by turning fat-soluble toxins into water-soluble ones so they can be excreted through your large intestine, kidneys, and skin. When you have a hormonal problem, however, your liver's function is compromised (often because your pathways of elimination are clogged). This means that your liver doesn't work as efficiently as it should and thus is unable to remove toxins as rapidly as they build up.

Your body copes with this problem by squirreling those fat-soluble toxins into—where else?—your fat tissue. For the moment, this protects your liver because it minimizes the toxic load there. The problem, however, is that it becomes even more difficult to shed weight. Your fat cells don't want to let go of those toxins, because your body knows that doing so would pollute your bloodstream and create a toxic environment for your organs, including your

Each day has four areas of focus:

Meal plan: *what to eat*

Focus on digestion: *how to improve your eating experience*

Getting to thriving: *short activities to help you
process what you are learning*

Clean sweep: *releasing the old and welcoming the new
in your physical environment and your body*

*heart and your brain. The end result? Your fat cells cling to the toxins and your
body clings to your fat cells.*

*Fortunately, there's a way to get your body to release its white-knuckled
grip on your fat: up your dietary and supplemental forms of intake of vitamin
A, vitamin B, and vitamin C, as well as sulforaphane and the antioxidant
glutathione—nutrients your liver needs to detoxify effectively. By helping your
liver do its job properly, you'll prevent those toxins from becoming backlogged
and wreaking havoc on your waistline. Here's how you can help achieve that:*

- *Fill your diet with plenty of vegetables from the brassica family: cabbage,
cauliflower, broccoli, brussels sprouts, and all kinds of kale. Try to sneak
at least one brassica-type vegetable into every meal throughout the day.
Add them to smoothies and juices that you make, too.*

- *Reach for lemons and oranges. Add fresh lemon to your water. However,
not **all** citrus will do—grapefruit contains an enzyme that impedes liver
detoxification, so avoid it while you're working on getting your liver back
into shape.*

- *Sneak caraway and dill seeds into as many meals as you can. Grind them
in a spice grinder (a coffee grinder works, too) and rub them on chicken,
fish, or other meats before baking, combine them with whole grains, or
add them to homemade salad dressings.*

Staying hydrated is extremely important during this cleanse. It supports your body's ability to flush out toxins and keep your bowels regular. Try to drink more water than usual, aiming for at least eight glasses a day. If this makes you feel cold or bloated, drink your water warm or hot. You can also add a little lemon to your water, as this will help with the detox.

Shopping List

Before shopping, consult with the daily meal plan so that you can purchase quantities and choices accordingly. (Not everything on this list is mandatory.)

A day or two before the cleanse, stock up on:

- green apples
- pears
- avocados
- grapes
- lemon
- fresh berries (and other fruit you like, but no melon—it causes water retention)
- baby greens
- bok choy
- dark-green leafy vegetables (kale, collards, mustard greens, spinach, broccoli rabe)
- tomato
- carrots
- onion
- scallions
- cucumber
- celery
- radish
- fennel (or other simple spring vegetables)
- garlic
- parsley
- olive oil
- apple cider vinegar
- white fish (cod, tilapia, haddock, etc.)
- salmon (preferably wild, no tuna)
- beans (cannellini, lentils, black-eyed peas, chick peas, etc.)

- brown rice (long grain only: plain brown, brown basmati, or brown jasmine)
- quinoa
- kasha (buckwheat)
- your favorite herbal and green teas (if you use sweeteners, use stevia, raw agave nectar or raw honey—they contain valuable enzymes)
- flaxseed meal
- your favorite nuts or nut butter (almonds, cashews, etc.)

- Fiber Smart by Renewlife, Fiber Fusion by Enzymatic Therapy, or other fiber supplement
- Chlorella tablets by Jarrow (optional but strongly recommended)
- Green Drink—freshly juiced or powdered (I recommend Kyo-Green)

Non-food items you will need:

- containers to transport food
- a journal (you may want to buy a fresh one to mark the occasion!)
- a nice washcloth for hot towel scrub or dry body brush

- Epsom salts or salt scrub
- a sharp knife and a mandolin for slicing
- a cutting board
- a soup pot

Preparation Day

Food Prep

It's important to spend a little time the day before your cleanse preparing your meals in advance, especially if you'll be keeping up with your normal work routine during the cleanse. That preparation will reduce the amount of time you spend in the kitchen during the four days and will keep things simple and accessible. One thing you definitely want to avoid is getting home after a long day to find there is nothing in the fridge ready to eat. That's not fun on a regular day, so imagine how you would feel while resetting. Read through the entire meal plan in advance and then use these preparation guidelines and recipes to get started.

What you'll need to prep for the first three days:

- **Fruit salad:** This will be breakfast every day, so feel free to chop apples in advance or make it as you go.
- **Liver cleansing medley:** I use the term "liver cleansing medley" instead of "salad" to emphasize the fact that this is much more substantial than just lettuce. You'll be eating this with every lunch, so make a big batch of any of the medleys listed below. If you keep the dressing separate and use a sealed container, it can last you all week long.
- **Grains:** Make a batch of brown rice or quinoa.
- **Protein:** Use the fish or bean recipes below. You'll be eating fish for lunch, or just beans if you are vegetarian.
- **Large pot of soup:** This will be your dinner for the first three days. Choose from the Quick Veggie Soup or Mung Bean Minestrone below.
- **Greens:** Choose any from the list below, following the recipes or just mixing them in with your soup.

On the next pages, I've included some recipes to guide you with the preparation, but feel free to improvise and add in your own ideas!

Mind Prep

This is your chance to really set your intentions for a new relationship with your body as you sync up with your WomanCode! Changing your food changes your brain chemistry and allows you to make changes in other areas of your life more easily. Take advantage of the lifestyle exercises I've included with each day specifically for that purpose. They are an essential part of the WomanCode Reset. Don't cheat yourself by just doing the food part and missing the life-changing messages that your body is trying to send you this week! The gift of these three days is clarity to create a new vision for yourself and your life.

Recipes

 SOUPS

Quick Veggie Soup

- *In a large pot of water, toss chopped garlic, onion, celery, carrot, parsley, and turnip.*
- *You may add any other leafy greens that you like: escarole, cabbage, and kale are great.*
- *Let simmer about 30 minutes, or until veggies are soft, then serve.*

Mung Bean Minestrone

- *Sauté 1 chopped onion in olive oil, salt, and pepper for a few minutes.*
- *Add a few chopped carrots and continue sautéing.*
- *Then add 1 quart of vegetable broth or water and cook until carrots begin to soften.*
- *Add 2 chopped zucchini and 2 chopped yellow squash, 1 can peeled crushed tomatoes (or fresh chopped tomatoes), and 1 bag frozen cut string beans.*

- *In a separate pot, cook mung beans (see recipe on page 123). Lentils make a fine substitution.*
- *Add beans to soup when finished.*

LIVER CLEANSING MEDLEYS

Fruit Salad (only for breakfast)

- *Chop and/or mix any combination of the following: green apples, pears, blueberries, blackberries, raspberries, strawberries, grapes.*
- *Squeeze fresh lemon juice on top and sprinkle with ground flaxseeds.*

Spring Mix Salad

- *Using a mandolin (or a regular knife—whichever you prefer), slice 1 bunch radishes, 1 cucumber, a few stalks of celery, and a few carrots (or other veggies of your choice).*
- *Mix in a bowl with mesclun greens and/or arugula and a jar of artichoke hearts, drained and sliced. Dress with olive oil and apple cider vinegar.*

Bok Choy Salad

- *Slice thinly and mix together: 6 stalks of bok choy, ½ small red onion, 1 Granny Smith apple, and (optional) ½ cup of sprouts. Add lemon juice, salt, and coriander.*
- *Veggies will get softer from the lemon juice/salt combo, so the longer you let it sit, the better it tastes! Dress with olive oil before serving.*

Raw Kale Salad

- Chop 1 bunch of lacinato (dinosaur) kale, thinly slice ½ red onion and a fennel bulb.
- Toss in a bowl, squeeze the juice of 2 lemons over the salad and sprinkle with salt. Let it sit for a few hours or overnight until it wilts (the longer, the better).
- Dress with olive oil before serving.

GREENS

Steam Sautéed Veggies

SUPER easy—for any of the leafy green veggies.

- Simply wash your greens under the faucet.
- Tear up leaves and discard the stems/stalks.
- Toss the greens into a sauté pan that has 1 tablespoon of oil in it.
- Heat through and sprinkle with sea salt.
- Wait 1 minute, then add ½ cup of cold water.
- Cover with a tight-fitting lid.
- About 5 minutes later, the greens will be perfect.
- Add any condiment you'd like (toasted sesame oil, olive oil, tamari, herbs and spices).
- Stir before serving.

Some examples with variations . . .

Sautéed Escarole

- Sauté ½ bunch of scallions in olive oil in a large pan.
- Add 1 head escarole chopped into small pieces, add a few splashes of water, cover for a minute, and cook until wilted.

Collards

- Sauté ½ chopped onion and 1 chopped red bell pepper in olive oil for a few minutes.
- Add 1 head collards, de-stemmed and sliced into thin strips.
- Season with salt, pepper, and nutmeg.
- Add some water, cover, and cook until greens are tender.

GRAINS

Basic Brown Rice Recipe

- Rinse 1 cup of rice in a colander.
- Add 1 tablespoon olive oil and rice to a pot and sauté for about 5 minutes until rice gives off a nutty aroma.
- Add 2 cups of water to pot and bring to a boil.
- Reduce heat to low and cover with a tight-fitting lid.
- Let cook for about 45 minutes, or until all water is absorbed.

Quinoa Recipe

- Rinse 1 cup of quinoa in a colander.
- Add quinoa and 2 cups water to a pot.
- Bring to a boil.
- Reduce heat to low and cover with a tight-fitting lid.
- Let cook for 15 to 20 minutes, or until all water is absorbed.

Spring Style Pilaf

- Cook 1 cup brown rice. Julienne radishes, and chop scallions and watercress leaves. Add brown rice vinegar and olive oil and toss all ingredients together.

PROTEIN

Lively Lentils

- *Place dried lentils, chopped onion, and chopped wakame (or other sea vegetable) in a saucepan. Cover with water. Bring to a boil, and then simmer until lentils get soft. Season with parsley.*

Magnificent Mung Beans

These beans are ideal for cleansing!

- *You may pre-soak them or, to soak in a hurry, pour boiling water over beans in a pot, let sit for 15 minutes, then drain and rinse.*
- *In a large pot, add 2 parts water to 1 part mung beans and a strip of kombu.*
- *Bring to a boil, then cover and simmer until beans are cooked fully.*

Easy Beans

For those of you without the time or desire to cook beans from scratch, I recommend using canned beans—Eden Organic is a favorite brand.

- *Try some great spring bean options: cannellini, black-eyed peas, lentils, and mung beans.*
- *Simply pop open the can, pour into a colander, and rinse.*
- *Eat them as is, adding spices and oils, or heat them up by sautéing with olive oil.*
- *Try adding chopped scallions or onions to give them a little flavor.*

SALMON AND WHITE FISH RECIPES

I recommend broiling, pan-cooking, or baking the fish "en papillote," a French style of cooking the fish wrapped in parchment, which keeps it from drying out (yum!).

Broil:

- Brush fish fillets with olive oil, lemon juice, and spices.
- Place fish on a piece of aluminum foil and put in broiler.
- Cooking times will vary, depending on how thick or thin the fish is.

Sauté:

- Heat olive oil in a frying pan.
- Add fish fillets and cook on each side for a few minutes.
- As when broiling, cooking times will vary, depending on how thick or thin.
- Season with lemon juice and spices.

En Papillote:

- Preheat oven (or toaster oven) to 400°F.
- Create an envelope pouch with a sheet of parchment.
- Lightly oil the paper and put fish fillet inside.
- Add some lemon juice, sliced veggies, and spices.
- Fold the parchment to close the envelope pouch, then wrap a piece of aluminum foil around everything.
- Place in oven and cook for 6 to 10 minutes.
- Be careful—it will be steamy when you open it up!

CLEANSE ENHANCERS

Green Drink

(with your breakfast or midmorning snack)

- *In a juicer—at home or at a health food store—juice 3 to 6 stalks celery, ½ cucumber, ½ cup parsley, ½ green apple, and 1 whole small lemon with skin.*

Immune Booster

- *Grate daikon radish (about 3 inches) and/or ginger root and/or 1 clove raw garlic chopped fine or pressed. Add to salads, veggies, or grains. These foods are anti-microbial and blood cleaners—they will give your immune system a real boost!*

Day 1: *Easing into It*

MEAL PLAN

● *Breakfast and/or Early Morning Snack*
- An 8-ounce glass of water
- Fiber supplement
- Fresh fruit salad with lemon juice (up to 1½ cups) and 1 tablespoon flax meal
- Green drink and/or Chlorella tablets

● *Lunch*
- Brown rice or buckwheat or quinoa with 1 tablespoon flax meal (up to ½ cup)
- Protein: 4 ounces salmon or white fish (no tuna, please); or ⅓ cup beans if you are vegetarian
- Liver cleansing medley (unlimited)

● *Midafternoon Snack*
If you need a snack around 3 or 4 P.M., try any or all of the following:
- Another serving of your lunch or dinner meal
- Veggies or fruits from the list
- Water
- Hot tea

Listen to your body. Does it really want food? Or is it really asking for something else, but food is your usual solution to keep it quiet? Listen.

● *Dinner*

• *Quick Veggie Soup (unlimited) or Mung Bean Minestrone (up to 1½ cups)*
Note: if you don't put greens in the soup, make sure to have cooked
greens (unlimited) on the side.

FOCUS ON DIGESTION

When you eat in a quiet environment and focus on your food, your body
devotes more energy to digesting the food and absorbing the nutrients. You
also enjoy the flavors and experience more, and therefore require less food
to have a satisfying experience.

• *At the office: Find a quiet place to eat; minimize talking, e-mailing,*
  and web surfing. Just eat and focus on your breathing and chewing
  (20 times per mouthful).

• *At home: Leave the TV off. Eat alone or acknowledge to your partner*
  or family that during meals you will be eating more slowly and
  talking less.

GETTING TO THRIVING

Tonight, take 10 minutes to write in your journal and get clear on your
intentions for this reset. What do you really want to get out of these four
days? This is your opportunity to get excited and think big. Don't let
thoughts of being "practical" get in your way here. What would really
make you excited in terms of results by the end of this time?

CLEAN SWEEP

Today find one thing you can throw out of your home, and I don't mean the trash! Find your edge. You know what you're holding on to. You know what you secretly have pack-ratted away. The space we live in reflects what's going on inside us, and it can get congested, just like we get congested in our bodies. The good news is, we can create change in our bodies by changing our outside environment! So, let's get started: Open your closet and find at least one thing—an article of clothing, shoes, sports equipment, or whatever—that you have not used in the last year. Give these items to the Salvation Army or to your neighbor—or just toss them. Create space for new and exciting things in your life. Life is dynamic—if we hold on to old things, new things will not fit in. Get that one thing in the trash by tonight. Don't put it off—tomorrow will bring a new assignment!

Use a dry brush before your showers while you cleanse and brush toward your heart for best results. Dry brushing provides your organs of detoxification a gentle internal massage to stimulate digestion. It also helps with your circulation.

Day 2: *Being Gentle with Yourself*

How's it going? By now you may be feeling lighter and more energized. You may also notice some headache or other discomfort. Either reaction is fine and normal, and you are taking the steps to ensure that your blood sugar stasis gets recalibrated, your liver gets a chance to be nourished, and your body can detox from estrogen.

MEAL PLAN

- **Breakfast and/or Early Morning Snack**
  - *An 8-ounce glass of water*
  - *Fiber supplement*
  - *Fresh fruit salad with lemon juice (up to 1½ cups) and 1 tablespoon flax meal*
  - *Green drink and/or Chlorella tablets*

- **Lunch**
  - *Brown rice or buckwheat or quinoa with 1 tablespoon flax meal (up to ½ cup)*
  - *Protein: 4 ounces salmon or white fish (no tuna, please) or ⅓ cup beans if you are vegetarian*
  - *Liver cleansing medley (unlimited)*

- **Midafternoon Snack**
  If you need a snack around 3 or 4 p.m., try any or all of the following:
  - *Another serving of your lunch or dinner meal*
  - *Veggies or fruits from the list*
  - *Water*
  - *Hot tea*

Listen to your body. Does it really want food? Or is it really asking for something else, but food is your usual solution to keep it quiet? Listen.

● *Dinner*

  • *Quick Veggie Soup (unlimited) or Mung Bean Minestrone (up to 1½ cups)*
  Note: if you don't put greens (unlimited) in the soup, make sure to have cooked greens on the side.

FOCUS ON DIGESTION

Increase your chewing at lunch to 15 chews per bite of food, 30 if you're well practiced. Notice that you produce a lot more saliva when you chew for longer, and that you can swallow the saliva without swallowing the food right away. Saliva is such an important element in our whole digestive process and we often just skip it, swallowing our food quickly and making our bellies do much more work.

Also, now that you've had one really light day on Day 1, start to pay attention to how this food feels going in your body. Notice how it feels to be eating less—how is your mental state?

GETTING TO THRIVING

Self-Care Reset: Spend some time journaling about the things that feel self-nurturing to you. Most of us assume self-care is expensive and indulgent. Instead, the most sustainable self-care comes from the little ways we can be compassionate to our bodies every day. For inspiration, think of things that your mother did for you or you do or would do for your own child. Brainstorm a few ideas and commit to doing one a day for the next week and see how you feel.

Don't let this assignment slide. Let this be the beginning of a beautiful, loving, and supportive relationship with your body!

CLEAN SWEEP

Did you throw out/donate one item last night? If you haven't already, please do that today. And add one more item that you are holding on to, but that you know has got to go.

However, the kitchen is our real goal for this evening: Please go through your spice rack/cabinet/ pantry and discard anything that has MSG, partially hydrogenated oils, and that is old. (You know you've had that chili mix for five years!) You also want to throw out any funky seasonings, marinades, sauces, or other nonfood items that are lingering around your fridge or pantry.

Instead, think fresh! Replace these items with good-quality sea salt, pepper to grind, and organic non-irradiated herbs and spices like cumin, turmeric, coriander, and thyme.

If you can, schedule a massage or an acupuncture session for tomorrow to relax and treat yourself. It can also help alleviate any detox symptoms you are experiencing.

Day 3: Clearing Out Any FLO Blockers

The focus for Day 3 is environmental stresses and toxins. As you reset internally, you may notice more how physically hard modern living can be at times. Pay attention to how you feel about the pace of where you live. What goes on for you, beyond the obvious "it's stressful"? What does the sensation in your body feel like? You experience this constantly, but when you are full of junk food, or just overstuffed, it's easier not to notice. Identifying how your body responds to environmental stress can be a key in eliminating binge and emotional eating. It's okay to feel your feelings!

MEAL PLAN

● *Breakfast and/or Early Morning Snack*
- *An 8-ounce glass of water*
- *Fiber supplement*
- *Fresh fruit salad with lemon juice (up to 1½ cups) and 1 tablespoon flax meal*
- *Green drink and/or Chlorella tablets*

● *Lunch*
- *Quinoa (up to ¾ cups) with 1 tablespoon flax meal*
- *Large liver cleansing medley (unlimited)*
- *½ avocado*

● *Midafternoon Snack*
If you need a snack around 3 or 4 P.M., try any or all of the following:
- *Another serving of your lunch or dinner meal*
- *Veggies or fruits from the list*
- *Water*
- *Hot tea*

Listen to your body. Does it really want food? Or is it really asking for something else, but food is your usual solution to keep it quiet? Listen.

- *Dinner*
  - *Quick Veggie Soup (unlimited) or Mung Bean Minestrone (1 cup)*
  If you don't put greens (unlimited) in the soup, make sure to have cooked greens on the side.

FOCUS ON DIGESTION

Today you're not having any animal protein, so really enjoy each bite of food at lunchtime. Sit back, look at your food, and notice the colors and textures. Breathe. Take the time before you eat to appreciate what you will be eating. When you heighten your awareness like this, you will naturally get more out of each mouthful. How does it feel to be vegan for one day? Notice how it feels to be eating less. It is normal to experience cravings and hunger and to not always indulge. How are your emotions?

EASE YOUR EXERCISE

When going through the WomanCode Reset it's normal that you may feel tired. You may also develop some constipation simply due to the smaller quantity of food that you're consuming. The very best thing you can do is stay well-hydrated and scale back on the amount of activity you plan to do this week. Try to rest when you can. Keep physical activity low to prevent exhausting yourself—instead of cardio boot camp, for instance, take a thirty-minute walk each day. Save the more vigorous activity for when you're done with the reset. If you're feeling very tired, but need your energy for an important appointment or meeting, take a vitamin B12 supplement for a boost of energy.

GETTING TO THRIVING

Tonight you should be doing very little.

Abundance assignment: Spend some time journaling about the things in your life that mean a lot to you. Then create a list of people who give you energy when you interact with them, who support you as you deal with stress in your life, and who support you being the best you. Brainstorm one thing that you can do to show each person how much they mean to you, spending little to no money. Get those creative juices flowing!

Don't let this assignment slide. Let this be the beginning of a more abundant life for you. We'll talk more about abundance tomorrow.

CLEAN SWEEP

How does your kitchen pantry look? How big was your bag of junk? We're curious to know, so write in to let us know your statistics! Take some pictures and share your new pantry with us!

Now we're moving on to the bathroom!

The products you use to clean your bathroom and household are potential stressors on your health. New scientific research shows that many of the chemicals found in everyday house-cleaning products are bio-accumulative and very toxic, which means that once in your system, they stay in your system and allow for increased free radical damage, which makes you more vulnerable to autoimmune diseases and cancers

Ready to throw things out now?

Find your bleach products, Comet, Ajax, Windex, Lysol, air fresheners, Glade Plug-ins, cute toilet bowl cleaners, and talc-based baby powder. Throw them in a garbage bag and toss them out.

What ever will I clean with?! No worries, here's a list of equally effective and bio-safe cleaning products:

- *Seventh Generation line of cleaning products: You can find this at some grocery stores, any health food store, and definitely Whole Foods.*
- *Orange Oil multi-surface cleaner: dishwashing liquid, laundry detergent, toilet bowl cleaner, and mirror cleaner, all in one. It's amazing and all natural.*
- *BonAmi or Arm and Hammer baking powder in place of Ajax or Comet.*
- *Hydrogen peroxide in place of Windex.*
- *White vinegar instead of bleach (plus it's a grease cutter for tile cleaning)*

Switching to these bio-safe products takes a load off your liver and helps protect your body year-round.

Day 4: *Using Your Body As a Tool to Create Your Best Life*

The focus for Day 4 is intentions and goal setting. Your reset is also creating mental and emotional clarity for you right now, so take advantage of this special time to set some goals for your New Year, starting right now with a meditation! Select two things that you want to have in your life that you don't have now. They can be objects, experiences, forms of support from others, positive beliefs about yourself, new behaviors, anything. Imagine these things or experiences in full, technicolor detail. Then describe exactly how these new things will change your life and exactly how you will feel when you have them. Be as specific as you can. Now imagine that these things and experiences are present in your life now. Feel the feelings of already having what you want. Notice any sensations of self-doubt or skepticism that come up and gently set them aside. Just breathe deeply and create in your body the feelings of already having these two things you've described. Hold on to those feelings for sixteen seconds. You are programming your body and mind to expect to receive these things into your life. By creating the internal experience of having or being something, you build subconscious confidence to actually pursue and achieve what you want with less effort and less self-sabotage.

How was your vegan day?

Are you doing a little less and resting more?

MEAL PLAN

- **Breakfast and/or Early Morning Snack**
  - An 8-ounce glass of water
  - Fiber supplement

- Fresh fruit salad with lemon juice (1 cup) and 1 tablespoon flax meal, plus 1 tablespoon nut butter or 2 tablespoons of nuts/seeds or ½ avocado
- Green drink and/or Chlorella tablets

● **Lunch**

- Brown rice or buckwheat (up to ½ cup) with 1 tablespoon flax meal
- Protein: 4 ounces white fish or 1⅓ cups beans
- Liver cleansing medley (unlimited)

● **Mid-Afternoon Snack**

If you need a snack around 3 or 4 P.M., try any or all of the following:
- Another serving of your lunch or dinner meal
- Veggies or fruits from the list
- Water
- Hot tea

Listen to your body. Does it really want food? Or is it really asking for something else, but food is your usual solution to keep it quiet? Listen.

● **Dinner**

- Small serving of quinoa (⅓ cup)
- Cooked dark-green leafy vegetables (unlimited), such as collards, mustard greens, turnip greens, spinach, etc., sautéed in or drizzled with 2 tablespoons extra virgin olive oil.

FOCUS ON DIGESTION

How are you doing with chewing? Eat S-L-O-W-L-Y. Remember to breathe while you eat. Notice how it feels to be eating protein. Notice the sensation of heaviness, notice how little protein you actually might need.

GETTING TO THRIVING

The Parable of the Leaping Cricket

> A small child put a cricket she had caught in her empty glass jar and screwed
> on the lid. The cricket jumped up and hit its head on the lid. It jumped a
> second time, and again hit its head. It jumped a third time, and realized there
> was no getting past this lid. From then on, the cricket only jumped half as
> high, never again bumping its tiny head on the lid of the jar. The child, feel-
> ing sorry about her game, took the lid off the jar and encouraged the cricket
> to jump out. But the cricket would not jump out. It jumped only half the
> height of the jar. The lid would always be there in its mind.

*Take the lid off your reality jar: What would your life look like if you dreamed
big and set goals to reflect your fantasies?*

*Take time tonight to think about what you want your life to be like this time
next year. What are your dreams? Hopes? What is the wildest and most
special thing that could happen for you in the next twelve months? Don't be
practical. Imagine yourself jumping high and peering over the lid of the jar.*

*Get out your old magazines and craft supplies and create a vision board
to reflect these dreams and visions for your future. Cut out images of all
that you'd like to see show up for you this year. Do you want a great job,
great home, loving friends and family, special items? Cut out images
that represent what you truly want and need in your life. (Use your old
magazines—and don't forget to throw them out after!) Using glue and
construction paper, make a collage and post it on your fridge. Look at this
collage daily, allow the images to program the reticular activator in your
brain, and trust that your vision is on its way to you now.*

*Also, write down some tangible, practical, proactive steps you could take to
accomplish these dreams. Who will you need support from? What will be
your biggest obstacles? What are you afraid of?*

The universe has everything in such abundance. It's all waiting for you. ASK!

CLEAN SWEEP

You've all done such a good job cleaning up your physical spaces. Now we want to focus on your insides. We've been decongesting the liver through this cleanse, but it's also very important to think about your bowel health, because this is where many of the old toxins and residues are actually processed out of your body once your liver has released them.

You should be having a bowel movement first thing in the morning without the aid of coffee or tea and another in the afternoon. If not, you are basically sitting with food that is days old.

So, if you have a tendency toward constipation, please:

> *Increase your water intake: have 8 to 16 ounces of water upon waking to get peristalsis going.*

> *Try a fiber drink. A favorite is Fiber Smart by Renew Life. It is made from ground-up flaxseed and oat bran, plus probiotics to ensure healthy intestinal flora levels.*

CELEBRATE!

What an amazing gift you've given to yourself—you should celebrate your commitment to health! Tonight, take a bath in Epsom salts and add your favorite essential oils. Your skin is your largest organ of elimination—heat helps pores open, and salt draws out toxins and impurities. So this bath is luxurious, but it also completes the detoxification you have been working on all week. If you aren't able to bathe, fill your sink with hot water and add the salts. Dip a clean washcloth in the water, wring out thoroughly, apply to dry skin and scrub yourself down.

We are here for you on e-mail or Facebook if you have any questions at all. Just write to us; we're here. What to eat after the reset? Hurry over to the next chapter to get the plan!

CHAPTER 5

From Vicious Cycle
to Delicious Cycle

In asking you to enlist your endocrine system—engage your WomanCode—as a partner in your health and healing, I'm actually suggesting that you do something much greater than that: I'm asking you to adopt an entirely new view of your health. For a slew of reasons (and FLO Blockers), many of us maintain a static mind-set about how our bodies should be. We believe that if our body performs at the same level each and every day, we've achieved a state of health, vitality, and success.

Yet what I've found is that it's against your very nature to be static; everything in your life, in your body, and in the world around you functions in a cyclical manner—from the seasons, to the moon, to your menstrual cycle, to your hormones, and so much more. To expect yourself to wake up feeling exactly the same way tomorrow morning as you did today is a misunderstanding of how forces in your body operate. Opening your eyes to this new, cyclical way of understanding your body may be the most profound thing you can do when it comes to repairing your relationship with your body. Harnessing this dynamic cycle allows you to enter into a state of FLO in your life. That's because, with the static view, when you expect your body to feel fabulous day in and day out, you continuously feel betrayed when it falls short. Not any longer.

Why is it so crucial to take this leap of faith and revise your mind-set? Because how you view your body determines the choices you make for it. If you're aligning with the cyclicality of your hormones, you'll make choices that respond to the cues your body is sending you. Your endocrine system does this cue-sending beautifully and predictably in an observable way that, if honored, will usher you toward a more efficient way of life.

Achieving your health goals becomes possible when you rely on your endocrine system for guidance. Living from this new place of cyclicality, on a day when you're feeling run down you might decide to take an easy thirty-minute walk instead of pushing yourself through a sweaty boot-camp class simply because you think that's what you *should* be doing. (Had you gone to that class, your tired body wouldn't have performed at the level you expected of it, leaving you feeling let down and depleted—not so after that soothing stroll.) In addition to tailoring your exercise in response to physical cues, you'll also make food choices that support your body instead of robbing it of energy. You'll develop a degree of sensitivity and attunement if your mind-set is one in which you believe things are meant to change. With that mind-set, it becomes your responsibility to adjust your daily regimen of food, exercise, sleep, and pleasure to respond to the daily and monthly cycles that occur.

In my own experience of healing, I found that enlisting my endocrine system to guide daily choices offered not only a greater opportunity for health, but also an extraordinary blueprint for optimal living in other areas of my life. Although my mind wanted to subscribe to a system that could potentially control all variables in my life, my body kept nagging at me that this wasn't in accordance with my nature. What was? Organizing myself, my life, my projects, my priorities, and my passions around my menstrual cycle. I call this my embodied time management. I knew that doing so would support my health; it would not put me in a position of setting up my life at the expense of my body, but rather would enable me to set it up in a way that would allow my body to flourish.

When I dropped the static view of my own health, I also let go of the static view of my career, relationships, and activities. After all, none of those things remain the same day in and day out either. In a word, the shift in mind-set was freeing. Instead of believing that achieving the same results in each category day after day equaled success, I saw that there was a natural ebb and flow to the elements of my life. And I realized that if I could organize my lifestyle under this context of cyclicality, I could get more done with less stress on my body and mind, and with greater ease, pleasure, and grace than I ever knew was possible. To me, that was the ultimate definition of success. This is also why I wanted to build a tool for women to take all the guesswork out of getting hormonally healthy and why FLOliving.com and the online hormonal improvement platform was born.

The WomanCode Protocol: Step 4—Syncing with Your Cycle for a Symptom-Free Future

Elite athletes and gym-goers alike know that cross-training is the key to optimizing physical performance while keeping injuries at bay. Whether you're a runner, cyclist, or swimmer, switching up your activity several days per week ensures that every muscle group gets both the work and the rest it requires to function at its peak. This is exactly what I'm suggesting that women need to do when it comes to the menstrual cycle, and doing so constitutes the fourth step in the WomanCode protocol. I call it cycle syncing—think of it as a form of embodied time management—where your hormones create structure. This practice comes back to the idea of using your body as a tool—harnessing your hormones to perform better, smarter, and more proficiently every single day. Doing so will also continue to heal your hormonal symptoms while preventing additional symptoms from developing.

To better understand how to sync with your cycle, it's first essential to learn what happens in your body during the four phases of your menstrual cycle. Let's take a look.

There are five hormones that govern your experience of your menstrual cycle: estrogen, progesterone, follicle-stimulating hormone (FSH), luteinizing hormone (LH), and testosterone. The quantities of these five hormones change four times throughout your menstrual cycle. This creates four distinct phases within each cycle— follicular, ovulatory, luteal, and menstrual—based on the concentrations of those hormones at each point. Not only do the varying ratios of hormones determine what's going on inside your body from a reproductive standpoint; they also determine how you feel physically and emotionally during each of the four phases.

Before explaining this to my clients, I ask them if they know what the four phases of their cycle are, and they often tell me they can identify two: the PMS phase and the bleeding phase. And you know what? They're not that far off from the truth. What's great about this response is that even if you haven't been consciously identifying where you are in your cycle at any given moment, you already know that changes occur from one week to the next. As you learn more about how to cross-train your life with your cycle later in this chapter, you'll be able to tune in to the subtler shifts that occur in your body each week and gain a deeper awareness of how the cyclicality of your hormones plays out on a physical and an emotional level.

Still, you may be wondering how the same cross-training approach can work for every woman, whether she's dealing with heavy periods, infertility, cystic ovaries, or any other hormone-based condition. The answer is this: because when you're coming at it from a *functional* standpoint and you're working with the endocrine system, it truly is a one-size-fits-all solution. The endocrine system functions in essentially the same way among all of us, so while the end result may differ based on the symptoms you're experiencing, you can harness the predictable cyclicality of your hormones to repair your condition now and prevent future hormonal issues in the future. This fourth step of the WomanCode protocol—syncing with your cycle—is the reason so many of my clients have improved their health so quickly, have stayed healthy, and have created a life they love.

The Four Phases of Your Menstrual Cycle

The four hormonal phases of your menstrual cycle are a blueprint for how to organize your life. Below, I'll show you how to zero in on what's happening with your hormones in each phase. I'll describe what's going on with your hormones and your body and outline the very best food, lifestyle, and physical activity choices to make in each phase. I've been using these skills with clients for well over ten years now, and I've found that it takes only about three months, on average, of consistently and consciously thinking about what your brain and body are primed to do during each phase before living in sync with your cycle becomes second nature.

☽ PHASE 1: Follicular Phase
Duration: 7–10 Days

- **Hormone focus.** The hypothalamus signals your pituitary gland to send follicle-stimulating hormone to your ovaries, telling them to get ready to release another egg. Several egg follicles start to swell in preparation. Estrogen increases to thicken your uterine lining so that it can host an egg.

- **Body focus.** Physical energy increases throughout this phase, and you may sometimes feel restless. Initially little to no vaginal secretions occur; then they start to increase—yellow or white in color and tacky or sticky in texture.

- **Lifestyle focus.** Creativity and new beginnings characterize this phase. This is the time to direct your energy into stimulating projects at work and at home. Plan brainstorming sessions with your coworkers; save your most mentally challenging assignments for this week, since your brain's penchant for creativity at this time makes it easier to problem-solve. Your physical energy is at one of its highest points during your follicular phase. Emotionally, you feel outgoing, upbeat, and revitalized. When setting your social calendar for the month, RSVP yes to invites during this week, when you'll have the most energy to be out and active. It's also an ideal time to plan to see a new exhibit or check out a new band: you'll be most open to the new experience and will find it most stimulating during this time.

- **Food focus.** Fresh, vibrant, light foods make you feel more energized during this phase, when all hormone levels are at their lowest. Your body can tolerate foods with a higher phytoestrogen content since, with estrogen just starting to increase, you won't be piling additional estrogen on top of already-elevated estrogen levels. Think: pressed salads (kimchi and sauerkraut), plenty of veggies, lean proteins, sprouted beans and seeds, and dense, energy-sustaining grains. How you cook your foods matters, too, so favor light cooking methods such as steaming or sautéing during the follicular phase. In addition, all of the recommended "Foods for Your Cycle" (see the chart on page 159 for the best foods to eat during *each* phase) are beneficial for improving ovulation that occurs in the next phase: avocados, for example, are known to improve the follicular-ovulatory transition as well as promote cervical mucus production.

• **Exercise focus.** Try something new—take that Zumba or yoga sculpting class you've been yearning to try at your gym. Putting your brain and body in a new, stimulating situation feels like an easy, natural thing for you to do at this time of the month. You also form new neuroconnections in the brain more easily, which means that stepping outside your comfort zone is a seamless thing to do; furthermore, new activities are more likely to stick when you start them now than at any other point in your cycle. You have the energy to go for those more challenging workouts at this time, too.

● **PHASE 2: Ovulatory Phase**
                 Duration: 3–4 Days

- **Hormone focus.** A sharp rise in follicle-stimulating hormone followed by an increase in luteinizing hormone, also from the pituitary, stimulates one follicle to swell further and burst, releasing an egg into one of the fallopian tubes; that egg then travels to the uterus. Estrogen levels continue to increase, further thickening the uterine lining and supporting the growth of immune system cells in the uterus. Testosterone takes a quick surge and drops right around ovulation.

- **Body focus.** Vaginal discharge increases and is clear, wet, slippery, or stretchy on your day of peak fertility. As you move past that peak day, vaginal discharge dries. You may feel pelvic pain with the release of the egg as well as a surge of energy or a sense of depletion, along with cravings or a headache.

- **Lifestyle focus.** Connecting with community is at the heart of this phase. This is the time to have important conversations, whether it's with your spouse, your mom, or your boss. If possible, hold off on having those conversations until this ovulatory phase, when your heightened communication skills will allow you to convey your thoughts and opinions more clearly, as well as to be more receptive to those of others. If you're planning to ask for a raise, do it during your ovulatory phase. This is also an ideal time to go on first dates, since your increased communication skills will make you that much more magnetic. And since you're at your most fertile in this phase, chances are (studies tell us) you put extra effort into looking and feeling your best in an unconscious effort to attract a mate when ovulating.

- **Food focus.** You have plenty of natural energy and your mood is stable because of all the estrogen floating around, so go easy on the carbohydrates and stick to lighter grains such as corn and quinoa. Still, you want to be sure your body is metabolizing and eliminating the surplus of estrogen efficiently, so fill up on veggies (the fiber aids elimination) and fruit (high levels of the antioxidant glutathione support the first phase of detoxification in the liver). The ovulatory foods (again, check out the "Foods for Your Cycle" chart) are about promoting vascular and antioxidative well-being for your ovaries so you can create the healthiest egg possible. These foods will also keep estrogen-driven symptoms, such as acne and bloating, at bay. Continue to focus on lighter preparations of foods, such as steaming or, when appropriate, eating foods raw.

- **Exercise focus.** When deciding which activities are best during this phase, keep two things in mind: high-impact workout and group settings. Your energy levels are at their max, so you're primed to take on more strenuous exercise such as weight lifting, plyometrics, and running. Since communicating and connecting with others also feels great on these days, consider running with friends or a team or taking swimming, dancing, or spinning classes.

☾ PHASE 3: Luteal Phase
Duration: 10–14 Days

- **Hormone focus.** The corpus luteum (the follicle from which the egg bursts) grows on the surface of the ovary, causing it to produce progesterone. The rise in progesterone signals the body to keep the uterine lining intact. It also signals the pituitary to stop sending out follicle-stimulating hormone and luteinizing hormone, ensuring that only one egg is released into the uterus at a time. Estrogen levels continue to rise. Toward the end of the cycle, if the egg hasn't been fertilized, the corpus luteum is reabsorbed into the body. Progesterone production will soon halt as a result, triggering your period. Testosterone will increase toward the end of this phase.

- **Body focus.** Physical energy declines, and premenstrual symptoms may develop toward the end of your cycle—symptoms such as bloating, irritability, headache, mood swings, and cravings.

- **Lifestyle focus.** Awareness, attention, and comfort are key now. As the corpus luteum is reabsorbed, your energy begins to soften and turn inward. You'll notice that you have the desire to nest, making the luteal phase an ideal time to take care of domestic chores, whether your list includes reorganizing your shoe closet, doing a month's worth of laundry, or making a big grocery-shopping trip. The particular ratio of estrogen to progesterone in this phase makes you notice things around you that you didn't see before. As a result, your brain begins to prioritize administrative detail-driven responsibilities you may have ignored all month, perhaps giving you the urge to clean your apartment from top to bottom, reconcile your online banking, or cook a week's worth of meals at one time. You'll also feel a need to nest on an internal level, perhaps paying extra attention to your self-care regimen, such as taking long, luxurious baths or simply relaxing with a book or a movie. Try slowing down social engagements during your luteal phase so you won't feel needlessly exhausted.

- **Food focus.** The foods you see listed for the luteal phase in the "Foods for Your Cycle" chart are rich in B vitamins, calcium, magnesium, and fiber. Combined, they will optimize the quality of the luteal phase in several ways. First, these foods stave off sugar cravings caused by the heavy use of B vitamins in promoting progesterone production. Second, the calcium-magnesium combination in leafy greens is essential in mitigating the effects of fluid retention that are so problematic for women during this phase. Finally, the fiber concentration will help your liver and large intestine flush estrogen more efficiently through the bowel, ameliorating the effects of estrogen dominance. In addition, healthy, natural sugars help with the dip in estrogen that occurs in the second half of the luteal phase and that can make you feel irritable. One of the best ways to achieve this is by roasting or baking vegetables, which increases the concentrations of those sugars so the veggies taste sweeter. In addition, make sure you have an adequate intake of complex carbohydrates to stabilize serotonin and dopamine levels in the brain and help prevent mood swings.

- **Exercise focus.** During the first half of the luteal phase your energy may still be high, so continue with the more strenuous activities you took on during ovulation. Then scale back on your intensity during the final five days with activities such as walking, Pilates, gyrotonic training, and vinyasa yoga. You may feel a little more sluggish and experience more water retention toward the end of this phase, so choose exercise with lower resistance (such as using the elliptical trainer)— you'll still be working your muscles, but it won't be as jarring for your body.

○ PHASE 4: Menstrual Phase
Duration: 3–7 Days

- **Hormone focus.** Progesterone production drops off as the corpus luteum disappears, triggering the shedding of your uterine lining in your menstrual phase, a.k.a your period/bleeding phase. Estrogen peaks and then drops, stimulating your hypothalamus to prepare for another cycle of ovulation.

- **Body focus.** A combination of brown spotting and red bleeding characterizes this phase. You may also experience pelvic cramping, low backache, fatigue, and cravings. Sometimes you may feel a sense of relaxation and relief as your estrogen peak passes.

- **Lifestyle focus.** Self-analysis and course-correction are dominant now. During your menstrual phase, the communication between the right and left hemispheres of your brain is more powerful than at any other time. This enables you to judiciously evaluate how you're doing in your life and, if necessary, begin identifying and making course corrections that will reposition you in the direction that you want to be heading. Because of the way your hemispheres are firing back and forth, you're also most likely to receive clear intuitive-gut messages during your menstrual phase. Check in. Listen to what those subtle messages are, especially if every month you're coming up against the same thoughts, worries, or fears at this time. Many women find that journaling during their menstrual phase, especially when they first learn to sync with their cycles, allows them to access deeper insight into what their instincts are telling them. It also helps them begin to notice thought patterns that may occur month after month, urging a particular action. Many women feel relieved when they learn that feelings such as restlessness and dissatisfaction during the menstrual phase are completely normal. Instead of allowing these thoughts to make you feel overwhelmed, take advantage of this phase to identify which areas of your life need your attention. Those messages will be most clear to you at this time. Then use the other weeks in your cycle to address these issues in a variety of different ways to help you come up with the best solutions and improvements for you.

- **Food focus.** During your menstrual phase your body is involved in an intense process—eliminating the lining of your uterus—so focus your diet on foods that add nutrients. As you can see from the "Foods for Your Cycle" chart, these include foods with a low glycemic index and water-rich fruits and vegetables. Seafood and sea-based veggies will also help remineralize your body with iron and zinc, which you lose during menstruation. The foods for the menstrual phase are all deeply restorative to the blood and kidneys—perfect for while you are bleeding. Choose whatever preparations feel most comforting to you. (Hint: for most of the year that will be soups and stews.)

- **Exercise focus.** Rest and recovery are important parts of any exercise program so that your body can repair. Schedule rest or yoga during the early part of the menstrual phase, especially the first day or two, when your flow may be heaviest. Take time to stretch and walk on these days. As you move into the end of bleeding and toward the follicular phase again, begin to amp up your activity according to how you feel.

Seeing Red: Interpreting Your Period

Variations in your menstrual flow can be excellent ways for you to see what's going on with estrogen and progesterone and gauge your overall hormonal balance. Give yourself a break from tampons at night so you can observe the quality of your flow.

Brown stains: If you period begins with a day or a few of this, it's an indication of some blood stagnation due to lower progesterone levels. When progesterone is low, you may also be noticing that your cycle doesn't start on time and though you may ovulate on time, your luteal phase is much longer than it should be. Vitex supplementation is excellent for this symptom.

Dark red or black clots: Large or small, this is another indication of lower progesterone, elevated estrogen, and congestion in the uterus. Dong quai is an excellent herbal support to reduce clotting, as well as uterine massage or acupuncture to help break up any adhesions that may be impeding blood flow.

Heavy bleeding: You go through a tampon an hour and a pad. You feel like you are bleeding out. This can be a sign of fibroids or polyps and it's

Syncing Your Cycle with Food

The food guidelines listed above and in the food chart (page 159) are based on three principles: food energetics, micronutrient support, and estrogen metabolism.

The concept of food energetics may be new to you. The idea introduced by Steve Gagné in his book *Food Energetics*, that different foods result in different energetic experiences within your body may seem "out there" at first, but it's actually quite intuitive. You feel drastically different when you eat roast chicken than you do when you eat a bowl of raw spinach, don't you? That's energetics—the fact that foods impart different energies within your body. The foods I recommend in each phase are aligned with the energy you experi-

important to visit your gynecologist to be examined. Focus on fiber here to help improve estrogen metabolism so the uterus is less stimulated during your cycle. Ward off potential anemia by eating plenty of beets to replenish your blood and supplementing with vitamin B12.

Short bleeding: Have you been feeling good about your period only lasting a day or two? It can indicate both extremely low estrogen and progesterone, which could be coming from key nutrient deficiencies and adrenal burnout. Get on a multivitamin and supplement with Omega-3 oil to supply your body with the key building blocks for hormonal output.

Very frequent bleeds: Do you feel like you're getting your period twice a month or all month long without a break? This is usually due to a sluggish thyroid and it would be great for you to have your thyroid levels checked to know what you're working with. Supplementing with a thyroid support complex like the one from Gaia Herbs is an excellent place to start, as it contains iodine and L-Tryosine, essential for the thyroid gland to have on hand to do its job properly.

ence and/or the kind of energy you need most to feel your best in each phase.

Next are micronutrients. Simply put, the foods in each phase provide your body with the building blocks it needs to support the hormonal ratios that occur in your body. You have different micronutrient demands depending on where you are in your cycle, and the foods in the chart at right deliver accordingly.

Finally: estrogen metabolism. You've already seen that estrogen levels vary from one phase to the next. And, as you know from earlier chapters, most symptoms that occur with hormonal conditions are due to an excess of estrogen within the bloodstream. Therefore, the foods in each phase are designed to keep estrogen moving through your organs of elimination and ensure that your liver has the support it needs to metabolize estrogen as efficiently as possible, detoxify it, and remove it from your body.

You may wonder whether you need to eat according to these principles 100 percent of the time to cross-train successfully. The answer is no. When you go to the grocery store, take this chart with you so you can front-load your diet with phase-appropriate foods the very best you can. As long as such foods make up the majority of your intake on any given week, it's okay if a portion of your diet comes from other parts of the list (depending on what you feel like and what's in season)—it's all great, healthy, endocrine-supportive food. And if you don't feel like having something roasted and heavy in the luteal phase because it's one hundred degrees outside, then by all means prepare the same recommended food in a way that feels more enjoyable to you. So start with the foods listed in the chart and do your best to create your meals around them. Given that this may require a big change in how you shop, cook, and eat, it may take some time before cross-training your life with food becomes second nature to you, your body, and your taste buds.

Why Cycle Syncing Works

Your menstrual cycle contains four distinct hormonal patterns. Each hormonal ratio changes your brain chemistry week to week throughout the month. Your neurochemistry is not the same from one day to the next, so why should you eat, behave, and move in the same way day in and day out? You shouldn't! That very premise of sameness doesn't allow you to channel your health and personal power as you could if you worked with what was actually going on in your body and your brain at the time. Each of the four distinct hormonal patterns within your menstrual cycle outfits you with different gifts and natural capabilities. Cycle Syncing means selecting behaviors that nurture you and engaging in activities that you can excel at based on what's going on biochemically and physiologically at that time. This includes:

- *Choosing foods that provide the nourishment you need at each point in your cycle.*

- *Choosing forms of exercise that honor and maximize your physical abilities during the four hormonal phases. This step of the protocol can support you if you aren't getting your cycle regularly due to menstrual issues like PCOS, as it can help regulate your cycle or, during the somewhat unpredictable transition of perimenopause, can help create a sense of stability, and can even be utilized after menopause to continue to engage your body cyclically. Women who have had hysterectomies or oophorectomies can even utilize the structure of this cyclical planning and embodied time management to regain their connection to their feminine biochemistry and to lunar cycles.*

- *Choosing tasks and activities—from cleaning out your closet to asking for a raise—that take advantage of what you're mentally and energetically poised to do because of your hormonal flux.*

SUCCESS STORY: *Emily Bohannon, 23*

CONDITION: Irregular, Painful Periods

About a year after moving to New York City, I started having two periods a month, sometimes menstruating for fourteen days at a time. They were incredibly painful, my emotions were all over the place, and my skin was breaking out like never before. I also often experienced bleeding during sex. As a result of all this bleeding, I was consumed with worry about my health. I consulted several doctors, and each gave the same answer: "I don't know what to do about this." I was confused, frustrated, and scared when a friend referred me to FLO Living.

My work with Alisa was nothing short of a miracle. I started feeling better after the very first session, and began to create a new dialogue with my body. Alisa is a wise and empathetic listener, and I felt wrapped in love and healing energy after every session. She introduced me to new, delicious foods and powerful supplements that helped my body return to its natural balance. We also addressed the ways in which my work and relationships were affecting my health. Most importantly, though, she gave me true peace of mind, and helped me get rid of my own judgment and shame about the messages my body was sending me. Alisa created a safe space and guided me gently into embracing and nurturing my feminine energy. By the end of my program, I felt juicy, alive, healthy, and more comfortable with my sexuality and body than ever before.

Through the WomanCode program, I now have one normal period per month, without any drugs. I don't experience the pain or emotional turbulence that I did before, and I've learned how to create healthy boundaries in my life to keep stress levels down. My skin is clear and gorgeous, and I enjoy nurturing myself with whole fresh foods (and the occasional cupcake, of course!).

WomanCode is the best thing I've ever done for my health.

Foods for Your Cycle

	Follicular Phase	Ovulatory Phase	Luteal Phase	Menstrual Phase
Grains	Barley Oat Rye Wheat	Amaranth Corn Quinoa	Brown rice Millet	Buckwheat (kasha) Wild rice

Vegetables	Artichoke
	Broccoli
	Carrot
	Lettuce: bibb,
	  Boston,
	  romaine
	Parsley
	Pea: green
	Rhubarb
	String bean
	Zucchini
		Asparagus
		Bell pepper,
		  red
		Brussels sprout
		Chard
		Chicory
		Chive
		Dandelion
		Eggplant
		Endive
		Escarole
		Okra
		Scallion
		Spinach
		Tomato
			Cabbage
			Cauliflower
			Celery
			Collard
			Cucumber
			Daikon
			Garlic
			Ginger
			Leek
			Mustard green
			Onion
			Parsnip
			Pumpkin
			Radish
			Squash
			Sweet potato
			Watercress
				Beet
				Burdock
				Dulse
				Hijiki
				Kale
				Kelp
				Kombu
				Mushroom:
				  button,
				  Shitake
				Wakame
				Water chestnut

Fruits	Avocado Grapefruit Lemon Lime Orange Plum Pomegranate Sour cherry	Apricot Cantaloupe Coconut Fig Guava Persimmon Raspberry Strawberry	Apple Date Peach Pear Raisin	Blackberry Blueberry Concord grape Cranberry Watermelon
Legumes	Black-eyed pea Green lentil Lima bean Mung bean Split pea	Red lentil	Chickpea Great northern Navy	Adzuki Black soybean Black turtle Kidney
Nuts	Brazil Cashew Lychee	Almond Pecan Pistachio	Hickory Pine nut Walnut	Chestnut
Meat	Chicken Eggs	Lamb	Beef Turkey	Duck Pork

	Follicular Phase	Ovulatory Phase	Luteal Phase	Menstrual Phase
Seafood	Fresh-water clam Soft-shell crab Trout	Salmon Shrimp Tuna	Cod Flounder Halibut	Catfish Clam Crab Lobster Mussel Octopus Oyster Sardine Scallop Squid
Other	Nut Butter Olives Pickles Sauerkraut Vinegar	Alcohol, moderate Chocolate Coffee Ketchup Turmeric	Mint Peppermint Spirulina	Bancha tea Decaf coffee Miso Salt Tamari

Below, you'll find some ideas of how to combine these ingredients to construct your WomanCode meals. **You can pick one from each meal or you could combine them all in smaller portions for each meal.** Trust your body to tell you what you might need and don't be

A Note on Soy

You may have noticed that I don't mention soy products very often. There is a reason for this. In my experience, women with estrogen-dominant conditions, like PCOS, fibroids, ovarian cysts, infertility, and low libido, have a harder time including this as a significant part of their diet. So often we tend to overconsume foods that are touted as health foods. Traditionally, Asian cultures consume no more than two teaspoons of fermented soy a day, which has been shown to be health promoting, while more than that quantity becomes problematic. Soy products contain high levels of phytoestrogens that mimic the body's natural estrogen hormones and if you're struggling to break down what you're already producing, adding more to your taxed system can make your symptoms worse.

afraid to experiment and get playful with your medicinal foods—these definitely won't hurt you! To access the recipes below, follow this link: www.FLOliving.com/cycle-sync-recipes.html.

Sample Day of Follicular Phase

BREAKFAST

- *Protein smoothie (using rice or hemp protein powder) with avocado, flaxseed, and cinnamon*
- *Oatmeal with cashews, goji berries, and cinnamon*

LUNCH

- *Poached chicken breast with parsley served with a sauté of broccoli, string beans, and carrots*
- *Lentil salad with chopped artichoke hearts*

DINNER

- *Omelette served with sautéed zucchini*
- *Romaine lettuce with sprouts, sliced avocado, and mung beans*

While small amounts of soy, especially those from fermented food sources—like natto, tempeh, soy sauce, and miso—have well-documented health benefits for women and their hormones, large concentrations of unfermented and highly processed forms of soy (tofu, soy burgers, soymilk, soy yogurt, soy ice cream, soy protein powder) can be problematic for two reasons. First, if they are GMO-based, research shows that this can be endocrine disruptive and can interfere with fertility in women and men. Second, they can inhibit thyroid function due to their high levels of goitrogens and the isoflavone genistein, which can be antagonistic to thyroid hormone. If you are vegetarian or vegan, you absolutely have other protein options available that are not endocrine disruptive, like eggs, seeds, lentils, or a variety of protein powders: rice, pea, and hemp.

Sample Day of Ovulatory Phase

BREAKFAST

- *Protein smoothie (using rice or hemp protein powder) with fig and coconut*
- *Quinoa flakes with pumpkin seeds and goji berries*

LUNCH

- *Quinoa salad with chopped greens and almonds*
- *Red lentil curry with turmeric over sautéed chard*

DINNER

- *Poached salmon with asparagus*
- *Endive and spinach salad with grilled shrimp*

Sample Day of Luteal Phase

BREAKFAST

- *Protein smoothie (using rice or hemp protein powder) with dates and mint*
- *Steamed sliced sweet potato with toasted walnuts*

LUNCH

- *Chickpeas sautéed with onion and cauliflower*
- *Brown rice with sautéed onion, carrot, celery, and daikon radish, topped with sunflower seeds*

DINNER

- *Roasted halibut with leeks*
- *Turkey tenderloins with sautéed cabbage and green apple*

Sample Day of Menstrual Phase

BREAKFAST
....

- *Protein smoothie (using rice or hemp protein powder) with dark berries*
- *Kasha with sunflower seeds and hijiki*

LUNCH
....

- *Miso soup, brown rice sushi rolls, and seaweed salad*
- *Sardines on toasted black rice bread with kale*

DINNER
....

- *Beet salad over steamed kale, with water chestnuts, hijiki, and shiitake mushrooms*
- *Mussels, squid, and scallops stewed in light tomato broth*

Cycle Syncing and Exercise

Have you ever felt like taking a yoga class, but talked yourself into going for a jog instead because it would burn more calories? Chances are the jog was ten times more difficult than it would have been if you'd *felt* like lacing up your sneakers from the get-go. Syncing with your cycle not only means respecting your hormonal patterns as you choose your foods; it also means listening to your body when it comes to the types of physical activities you do. During the first half of your cycle—the follicular and ovulatory phases—your energy is high. This is when the high-impact, challenging activities feel easiest—things like running, kickboxing, weight lifting, and spinning.

But during the second half of your cycle—the luteal and menstrual phases—your energy ever so slightly shifts and turns slightly inward.

This is the time to sign up for yoga and Pilates classes, spend a while at a consistent clip on the elliptical, or do other kinds of light cardio exercise, such as walking or riding your bike. You may find that you're too restless to make it through a vinyasa class during the first half of your cycle, but it's exactly what your body craves during the second half. Listening to your body and adhering to your own hormonal blueprint is much more intelligent, from an endocrine standpoint, than doing something you think you *should* do just because it's the latest trend. Not only will you get more out of the types of exercise that fit your hormonal reality, but—because your body is better equipped to do particular activities at particular times—you will be less susceptible to soreness and injury.

As you transition to a new perspective of cyclicality, I would ask that you give yourself some grace. If until now you've believed that you shouldn't feel any different throughout your cycle and regularly pushed yourself to do certain activities even when you didn't feel like doing them, it may take some mental and physical attunement to begin to look at exercise from this new standpoint of syncing with your cycle. But there's plenty of payoff for you to reap hormonally and physically. The *totality* of the different types of physical activity recommended above for each of the four phases of your cycle results in an incredibly well-rounded plan that challenges your entire body in different ways based on what your body requests that you do each week. In a thirty-day period you'll fit in strength, cardio, and flexibility training as well as rest. You'll prevent injury and forestall the internal stress that results from doing the wrong activities at the wrong times—stress that can ultimately threaten your endocrine balance.

The Stepping-Stones of Syncing Your Cycle

What's particularly satisfying, if you allow your hormonal patterns to lead, is that you'll get to do everything in a harmonious, enjoyable way. You'll reap the benefit of doing a variety of activity, but at no expense to your body, reproductive health, social commitments, career, sanity, or emotional well-being. I've mentioned before that cross-training your life doesn't happen overnight. If it feels daunting to you at first, please don't worry. It's an ongoing process you'll experience: you'll start with what feels most natural and pleasurable to you, and with each cycle you'll become more and more adept at making the best choices for your hormonal health.

Here's a look at the different stages you can expect to experience at your own pace as you learn to cycle-sync:

- *Stage 1: Observation and familiarization.* The first stage involves observing yourself in real time and noting your hormonal fluctuations in each of the four phases. You'll get to the point where you're able to know exactly where you are in your cycle simply by noticing your body's distinct cues.

- *Stage 2: Practice and adoption.* You start to layer in the food choices that align with the phase you're in and put into practice some of the lifestyle and exercise recommendations. Over time, you plug in more and more of the phase-specific food, physical activity, and lifestyle guidelines as they start to feel easier and more natural with every cycle.

- *Stage 3: Mastery.* This is where syncing with your cycle becomes second nature for you. It's the mind-set of, "This is where I am in my cycle, and this is what I must do to maintain hormonal harmony." You're able to anticipate things going on

Plan My Life Around My Period? Really?

If you're wondering whether it's truly possible to plan your life around your period, trust me: I understand where you're coming from. The key to wrapping your mind around this significant life change is to realize that I'm not asking you to go from one black-and-white view (the body is static) to another (the body works in a cyclical way that you must strictly adhere to no matter what life throws your way). Embracing a cyclical relationship with your body requires a commitment to flexibility and going with the flow.

*At first, cross-training your life may seem strange and almost overwhelming; going back to a lifestyle of ignoring your hormones may seem like a much easier way of life. But, as you already know, your hormones won't ignore you. If you choose that second approach, they'll send a message loud and clear to let you know they're being neglected. The key to making the first approach, cross-training, work is to look at the different recommendations in lifestyle, diet, and physical activity and turn up the volume on what you can do comfortably given what's going on in your life at the time. So maybe the first month you commit to stocking your refrigerator and pantry with the ideal foods for each phase and eat most of your meals according to your cycle— and that's **all** you worry about. Then the next month perhaps you layer in the exercise component. And the month after that perhaps you plan some phase-appropriate activities each week. There's no need to try to do it all at once. Rather, look at your life and what parts of cross-training feel most natural and pleasurable to you, and continue to build your experience, month by month, from there. The opportunities expand even into how you choose to interact with others in your life at ideal times and in ideal ways—whether that be with coworkers, romantic partners, or your own children.*

in your life that could threaten your sense of balance and then look for ways to minimize the potential impact they may have. (You'll read more about how to do this in chapter 6.)

When you sync with your cycle, you set yourself up with much better health, nutrient variety, and estrogen management, and with a much safer relationship with physical activity. You'll get more done without trying to do it all at once. The very nature of this new approach to your cycle and your life is that it safeguards the health of your period, fertility, and libido and helps clear up symptoms you may have in any of those three areas.

Rebuilding Your Relationship with Your Body

I was never looking for the menstrual cycle to be the holy grail of my life. I came at this strictly from the standpoint of needing to heal myself physically. But what I found from honoring the four phases of my cycle, and what I see in the women I work with every day who learn these same skills, is that doing so gives a woman access to so much more than a healthier, more fertile, more energetic body. Women who partner with their hormones live more efficiently and strategically. These women end up becoming the fullest expression of themselves and live as leaders and change-agents in their own lives and communities.

But the changes you'll make require so much more than simply following my protocol for what to eat, what to do, and how to live in each of the four phases of your menstrual cycle. For this plan to be successful, and to truly heal your castaway condition, it must become an effortless part of your monthly experience; and that requires a fundamental paradigm shift in the current relationship you have with your body. Let's face it: many women would rather exist from the neck up and would prefer their bodies take care of themselves. (Worse yet, many women believe that to be successful in their career, this is exactly what they *need* to do.) And yet the hormonal breakdown that results from ignoring your WomanCode is very likely what led you to pick up this book in the first place. That's why I want to make it clear: living in sync with your weekly flux will actually bolster—not deter—your career success. That's because you'll be leveraging your mental and physical abilities week by week to work more cleverly and seamlessly instead of pushing against your hormonal current every step of the way.

After living within this habit of syncing with my cycle for several years, I began to see even more profoundly how well it fits, not just with my body's natural rhythms, but with how my brain is designed,

Cycle-Syncing If You're on the Pill

Can you still sync up with your cycle if you're on the Pill? The answer is yes, but you'll do it in a slightly different way than a woman who isn't on the Pill. That's because hormonal contraception shuts down the processes that occur in your four phases. Specifically, you don't have a follicular phase and you don't ovulate. When you're on the Pill, synthetic hormones biochemically trick the hypothalamus, pituitary gland, and ovaries into thinking you're pregnant. As a result, you don't have most of the body cues, such as changes in cervical fluid, that a woman not on the Pill would have. But that doesn't mean you can't cycle-sync. In fact, it is a phenomenal thing to do no matter what; you'll reap the benefits that come from consuming a wide variety of foods, doing different kinds of exercise throughout the month, and making wise, varied lifestyle choices.

Here's how you do it:

• *Map out on a calendar when you finish the last day of your period.*

too. Women's brains, I learned, function more holistically than men's brains—that is, with a richer conversation between the left and right hemispheres. As a result, we synthesize multiple pieces of data simultaneously and feel better when we're integrating many different aspects of our lives at once. Men's brains, on the other hand, function in a more binary fashion—each man is more dominantly right brain or left brain. That's why it seems easier for men to live their lives in a rather linear fashion, while women require a life in which we're constantly synthesizing and integrating pieces of information.

This reality of synthesis and integration can seem overwhelming and complex, which is why I was completely inspired when I discovered that syncing up with my cycle meant that I could leverage my hormones and brain behavior and be incredibly productive and efficient. That's because I could continue juggling multiple tasks and

- *Consider the next day the first day of your follicular phase. Follow the follicular phase guidelines for seven days.*

- *The next day is your first day of the ovulatory phase. Follow the ovulatory phase guidelines for four days.*

- *The next day is your luteal phase. Follow the luteal phase guidelines for twelve days.*

- *The next day is your menstrual phase. Follow the menstrual phase guidelines for five days.*

- *Begin again with your follicular phase.*

My hope is that you'll notice the enormous rewards of syncing with your cycle even without all of the hormonal changes, and then, due to that preliminary success, wonder what it would be like to have access to all the physical and neurochemical opportunities your cycle delivers each and every month. From there, if you like, you can work with your physician to come off the Pill and begin to sync up with your cycle in a more comprehensive way.

opportunities—except now, rather than attempting to do all of them at one time, I could accomplish them all over the course of one month. I could take on certain tasks at certain points in my menstrual cycle—in other words, at those times when it was most natural for me to do them, based on what phase I was in—instead of struggling against my brain's hormonal reality.

So my goal isn't only to dazzle you with how cool your menstrual cycle is and how much more you can accomplish when you honor each unique hormonal phase. What I've experienced from women who use this program is that they realize they've been walking around thinking that their body is weak, vulnerable, out of control, and messy when it's not. It's nearly impossible to grow up in this culture without some of that residue on you. But for you to work with this protocol long term, I want you to make a new commitment—a commitment to work with, not against, your hormones and to leverage them for optimal health and happiness.

One-on-One with Alisa

Now that you've learned this entirely new way of going about your life, my hope is that you're excited to see what kinds of results cycle-syncing can create for *you*. Sit down and put your very first cycle-syncing calendar together. Identify where you are in your cycle now, and map out each of the four phases. Absolutely visit FLOliving.com to learn more about getting in sync with your hormones with the online program. Begin putting into practice the first four steps of the WomanCode Protocol with all the information you know now about the best diet, exercise, and lifestyle activities to engage in during each phase. You will set up the healthiest hormonal environment for your body to have easy periods, optimal fertility, and juicy libido!

CHAPTER 6

Life Happens—WomanCode Survival Strategies

At this point in your journey you've completed the first four steps of the protocol. When it comes to syncing up with your cycle, step 4, you've transitioned through the first two stages—observation and adoption—and you're moving toward the third and final stage of mastery. In this stage, you're able to go with the flow and adeptly respond to the changes that occur in your life from a place of honoring your hormones.

To move more deeply into this place, keep two important points in mind. First: your job, for life, is *always* to be thinking about how you can cross-train your life with your hormones—how you can front-load your body with the nutrients it needs in each phase, exercise in ways that respect your physical realities, and optimally plan your lifestyle to respect both your endocrine system and your obligations. The second aspect of moving more deeply into a state of hormonal mastery is listening to the conversation your endocrine system is having with you, on a daily basis, in the form of physical symptoms;

that conversation will help you understand how well you're doing each day. From there, you can determine whether you're on the right path and should keep doing what you're doing, or evaluate what's causing your symptoms and determine what adjustments you need to make in your diet, exercise, and/or lifestyle.

These two key points—syncing up with your cycle *for life* and regularly checking in with the cues your endocrine system is sending—make up what I call the dynamic equation. It's where your WomanCode meets your FLO. While cycle-syncing deals with the choices you make based on where you are in your cycle from one week to the next, the dynamic equation layers in what's going on in your everyday life to help you make the best choices possible for your body. When you engage the dynamic equation every single day, you move toward a place of becoming your own health coach. And from this place, not only will you prevent a total relapse of symptoms, but you'll also be in a position to prevent any future hormonal breakdown, because you're managing your hormonal health *on a daily basis*. As your own health coach, your role is to constantly work toward managing your dynamic equation in order to keep your hormones in a state of balance.

Above all, living the WomanCode way means being an active participant in your life. The whole point, after all, is to help your hormones reach their "happy place" so that you can engage in life even more fully. But how can you do this without feeling utterly deprived at every Starbucks-studded turn? How can you say yes to opportunities to celebrate and connect with friends without sending your entire endocrine system for a loop?

In this chapter, I lay it all out for you, starting with how to maximize your hormonal health on a daily basis using the dynamic equation. I'll also show you how to get your endocrine system back on track immediately after coming into contact with short-term FLO Blockers (endocrine disruptors) such as skipped meals, sugar-laden treats, boozy nights out, and much more. While my hope is that you'll do your very best to avoid these things, I also want to ensure that you have the skills necessary to prevent the potential hormonal disturbances that FLO Blockers can create if you get off track. Finally, I'll give you the tools you need to respond to situations that inevitably occur throughout the year—vacations, busy times at work, parties, and family gatherings—to minimize the impact they have on your short- and long-term health.

Cue the Hormonal Music

I've mentioned many times before that the endocrine system is predictable: it functions in a predictable way when things are working well, and it breaks down in a predictable way when things go awry. That's why the same functional approach to healing hormonal problems works from one woman to the next, no matter what their conditions may be.

But why is it so predictable in the first place? Credit Mother Nature. The endocrine system evolved to allow our bodies to maintain homeostasis in every imaginable environment. Simply put, that system strives to keep us functioning no matter what's happening *outside* our bodies—whether we're in the Arctic, the desert, or an air-conditioned apartment, whether we have an abundance of food or a shortage, and even whether we have massively stressful moments. What's more, our endocrine systems are so adaptable to ultimately safeguard our reproductive capacity and thus safeguard the survival of our species. Can you imagine what it would be like if the process of reproduction were different for each of us? It would be impossible to keep the human species going generation after generation. Since all of our endocrine systems work in the same way, the process of reproduction can occur through exactly the same series of events from person to person.

With this predictability in mind, our endocrine system sends us all the same signals when there's a problem somewhere along the line. As wonderfully unique as you are, the fact that you feel sluggish, cranky, and headachy when your blood sugar is low is as predictable as gravity. Being able to notice those cues, identify their cause, and make the appropriate adjustments constitutes the second part of the dynamic equation. Throughout this journey, as you've adopted the first four steps of the WomanCode protocol, you've built a much stronger relationship with your body and are now more aware of these signals than ever before. But I want to take all the guesswork out of it for you and help you identify which part of your endocrine system—blood sugar, adrenals, elimination, or reproductive organs—is waving the red flag. This way you can put the skills you'll learn later in this chapter into action in order to counterbalance the effects you're experiencing.

Let's look at the red flags—the warning signs—for each part of the endocrine system in turn:

Blood Sugar

- *High blood sugar.* Hyperactivity, jitters, dizziness, anxiety

- *Low blood sugar.* Headache, shaking, sweating, irritability, fatigue

Adrenals

- *Overworked adrenals.* Inability to concentrate, low physical stamina and endurance, low blood sugar symptoms, difficulty getting out of bed, hangover-like feelings when you wake up, insomnia, depression, anxiety, low libido, difficulty concentrating, poor memory, low immunity

Elimination

If you have congested pathways of elimination, you'll typically develop symptoms in the order that the organs of elimination are listed below. In other words, if you have signs of congestion at the level of the skin, the *final* organ listed, then everything before it is also backed up; so make sure you're taking the right actions to support *those* pathways to help resolve your skin issues. (See instructions in chapter 4 for supporting the various organs of elimination.) Conversely, if you experience symptoms related to the large intestine and leave those symptoms unaddressed, over time you'll experience a flare-up of symptoms in the liver, then lymph, then skin.

- *Large intestine.* Constipation, diarrhea, IBS, bloating

- *Liver.* Food sensitivities and allergies, pain (sharp or dull) under the right rib cage after eating a rich meal or drinking alcohol, sweating, foul body odor (especially from the armpits and feet)

- *Lymph and skin.* Acne (cysts, whiteheads, blackheads), rosacea, eczema, dandruff, oily scalp, body odor

Reproductive Organs

- *Signs of imbalance.* Physical cues that don't align with those described in the four phases of the menstrual cycle outlined in chapter 5, indicating that your estrogen and progesterone levels aren't balanced

Remember that symptoms of any hormone-based problem with your reproductive organs—problems such as fibroids, endometriosis, PCOS, and heavy/painful/missing periods—may stem from an issue in any of the other categories listed above as well. Fortunately, the WomanCode protocol will address these symptoms no matter where the problem first originated.

Your Health: The Ultimate Experiment

I sometimes have clients who log in for a session with me riddled with the guilt of going "off protocol" and ready to confess, but worried to disappoint. When they finally admit that they haven't been staying on track as much as they'd like and get the guilt out of their system, they are typically surprised by my response, which is usually: "Great!" I immediately want to know what symptoms they're able to observe, what triggered the slide, and how it made them feel. As far as I'm concerned, it's all research in partnering with the body. One of the many things you start to notice when living the WomanCode way is that the cleaner you eat and the more you remove FLO Blockers from your life, the more you become aware of what happens in your body when you do encounter those obstacles. (Remember the four FLO Blockers, a.k.a. endocrine disruptors, from an earlier chapter? They include misinformation about your hormones, cultural conditioning, toxic chemicals/products, and a hormonally disruptive diet.) When you get off course, when you succumb to FLO Blockers, the unpleasant results reinforce why you stuck with the protocol in the first place and make you feel more motivated to make healthy decisions at every meal, every day. Living the WomanCode way isn't an intellectual exercise about what you should be doing. Rather, it's what you *want* to be doing because you're partnering with your body to feel the best that you possibly can. Simply put, feeling good becomes a whole new currency in your life, and it's worth banking on.

A huge piece of setting yourself up for success and avoiding FLO Blockers, at least at first, is getting intimate with those FLO Blockers when you encounter them. Notice what they are and how they make you feel. What changes do you experience on a physical, mental, and emotional level? Before you ever knew what WomanCode meant, you may occasionally have felt bloated, gassy, and lethargic, but had no idea why. Now you might notice that you feel those symptoms after eating a greasy meal at a restaurant. Because you're equipped with the tools and awareness to connect the dots between what you ate and your tummy trouble soon after, you can use that knowledge to make cleaner choices the next time you go out to eat.

Recent scientific research reveals that focusing on your short- and long-term health goals (such as beating bloat, priming your body for a baby, or warding off disease) makes it easier to quash cravings and resist temptations. In a study published in the journal *Proceedings of the National Academy of Sciences,* researchers found that participants who focused on their health goals while experiencing a craving showed increased activity in their prefrontal cortex—the rational, decision-making part of the brain. When the prefrontal cortex is activated, it pulls the brakes on the reward system—the part of our brain that tells us to do things that feel good even if they're not good for us—because the two areas cannot fire simultaneously. The result: participants experienced a decreased desire for the treat. According to the researchers, this response is rather like a muscle. With practice, as with physical exercise for muscles, the more you focus on your health goals in the face of temptation, the quicker your prefrontal cortex jumps into action, and thus the easier it becomes to resist. On a psychological level, what I've observed over the past decade in myself and my clients is that it doesn't necessarily work to try to avoid all indulgent things and be perfect at all times. What does work: experiencing both the positive and negative results of your behaviors, because it's so much easier to make *positive* choices when you've fully felt the *negative* effects.

The more you're able to tap in to how your body feels based on what you feed it and what you do with it, the more you'll start to see the spillover into other areas of your life. Where better than in the bedroom? If you've been subsisting on caffeine and bagel fumes all day, running on little sleep, and trying to pack more into your day than you reasonably could into a week, you're going to crash into bed when you finally get home at night. If you happen to get intimate with your partner, your expectations when it comes to sex and what you're going to feel are going to be bottom-of-the-barrel low, given your energy level. You'll consider yourself lucky if you climax at all. There may even come a point when you wonder how much longer it'll last so you can finally go to sleep.

But what if the opposite were true? You powered your body with lean proteins, healthy fats, robust vegetables, and whole grains all day. You plowed through your to-do list with a calm mind and even had time for a workout. If you relax onto your pillow-top mattress after a bath after *that* sort of day, you're going to feel fresh and energized no matter how many hours you've been up. Not only are you going to be more sensitized to the positive effects you're experiencing in your body; you're also going to be more tuned in to the sensations you feel during sex. You're going to breathe more. You're going to relax more. You're going to feel your partner's touch on every inch of your skin. Not only can you expect to climax; your body and mental state are primed to have several orgasms—each bigger than the last.

That's what living the WomanCode way looks like: every positive behavior throughout each day adds up to a life of feel-good moments.

Managing Your Dynamic Equation

Like a good leader, you should always be prepared. When life happens and something disrupts your hormonal harmony, you'll want to know exactly what you need to do to get back in balance. The problem many women face when they encounter one slipup in their day is that they assume they've blown the *whole* day and let themselves get wildly off track from there. This, of course, makes it so much harder to find their way back. Clearing away an all-or-nothing mentality is the very first place to start, and it's one of the most freeing things you can do for your body and your health.

In my experience working with clients, I've come to see that there are predictable daily and annual situations that can threaten to disrupt your hormonal balance. First, let's tackle the **daily** trials and tribulations. I'll show you what you can do, when they occur, to counterbalance their effects. This will minimize the impact they have on your hormonal health. You'll see that most of the daily challenges are food-related. That's because, as you've learned, what you eat has a tremendous effect on whether your hormones function optimally or topple beneath a sugary pile of cupcake frosting. After all, there are hormone-disruptive food temptations all around you. Given those temptations, I'll show you what you can do from a diet, exercise, and lifestyle standpoint to reclaim your hormonal health when you *do* get off course.

Next, I'll address the **annual** (or sporadic) situations that arise in most people's lives and can put your endocrine system in jeopardy:

vacation, busy times at work, excessive drinking, and family gatherings. Unlike the daily situations I mentioned earlier, which can be somewhat unpredictable, you can mentally prepare for these events—and it's important that you do so. As you learned in chapter 5, where I explained how crucial it is to move from a static mind-set of your body to a cyclical mind-set, how you view your health has an incredible impact on the choices you make for yourself each and every day. So when it comes to these events that are guaranteed to pop up throughout the year, the mind-set you apply going in to each one will determine how well, hormonally, you emerge from it. And if you do slip up, you'll be able to catch yourself earlier and begin to engage the tools in the following section to rebalance your endocrine system.

Still, I completely understand the temptation to let yourself go during these events (hello, vacation!) and worry about cleaning up the hormonal mess afterward. Unfortunately, your hormones don't work that way. Since these occasions occur throughout the year, as soon as you've cleaned up the mess from one event, another will arise and send you backsliding all over again. This is the very thing I want to help you prevent. I want you to achieve a consistent state of health instead of forever running around the hamster wheel of getting healthy and unhealthy. If you're truly trying to accomplish whatever goal brought you to this book in the first place—whether it's improving your cycle, getting pregnant, or restoring your libido—it's crucial to enter into difficult situations with a mind-set that will yield the very best choices for your body.

✛ Your Daily WomanCode Survival Kit

Bouncing Back from Everyday Endocrine Disruptors

Endocrine Disruptor: SKIPPED MEALS

Between walking the dog, remembering to put on both earrings, shuttling your kids to school, and showing up for your morning meeting—which, by the way, you're leading today—your lips won't see a morsel of food until well past 10 A.M.

Managing the equation. Prevent a total blood sugar crash and ward off sugar cravings throughout the rest of the day.

Food. Grab emergency fuel—down a protein-based shake (buy bottled, such as Dole Fruit Smoothie Shakers or Special K Protein Shake, or keep single-serve packets of meal replacement shakes in your desk that you can mix with water when needed). This solution is not ideal, but it will keep your blood sugar from dipping to dangerously low levels. At your next opportunity to eat, have a combination of protein, fat, and carbohydrates, such as two slices of turkey breast, half an avocado, and brown rice.

Exercise. After you eat lunch, do ten squats over your chair. When you wait too long to eat between meals, your body goes into starvation mode and is more likely to store glucose as fat at your next meal. A short bout of exercise will help your muscles burn some of the glucose for fuel to reduce the total amount of sugar in your bloodstream.

Lifestyle. Say no to after-work commitments. Instead, go home and put that time toward preparing a proper evening meal, and make sure you have breakfast ready for the next day to prevent a recurrence of *this* morning. Use your evening to prepare make-ahead foods such as hardboiled eggs (they last a week in the fridge), to prepack smoothie ingredients for throwing into the blender in the morning, or to cook a batch of oatmeal to heat up in the A.M.

....

Endocrine Disruptor: **EXCESS SUGAR**

It's the third office birthday party of the week. You successfully avoided the cheesecake at Rachel's and steered clear of the ice cream social for Bob's, but your resolve fades when you come face to face with the pillowy strawberry-frosted vanilla cupcake at Lynn's—and maybe you'll have just a taste of the coconut and a sliver of the key lime, too.

Managing the equation. Avoid stressing your body out with the influx of sugar and minimize your body's physical response to food sensitivities (such as those to the gluten found in wheat). In addition, keep your bowels moving to remove all of these processed food substances, which threaten to slow down transit time and potentially increase estrogen in your bloodstream.

Food. Take a dose of a B-vitamin complex supplement to take some of the strain off your adrenal glands, which may be overreacting to the sugar trip. Take a dose of quercetin, an anti-inflammatory that calms your body's inflammatory response. At your next meal add two tablespoons of flaxseed to speed up transit time. Stir it into vegetables, soup, salad, or grain. Be sure to eat something loaded with healthy fats as well, such as a handful of nuts or a scoop of natural peanut butter, to stabilize your blood sugar.

Exercise. After work, do a high-intensity interval training routine on the treadmill: walk at a brisk clip for two minutes, sprint at your max for thirty seconds, and return to walking briskly for two minutes. Repeat for a total of twenty minutes.

Lifestyle. Share your health objectives with your coworkers—tell them about the changes you've been making and the differences you've experienced so far. They'll learn why it's important for you to stay on track and may start bringing healthy options (such as fruit salad that *everyone* can enjoy) to parties. When others know about your health goals, you'll also be more likely to stick with them—and less tempted by treats—because you'll feel more accountable for your actions. In the evening, shut off all stimulation, including TV, computer, cell phone, and tablet, by 10 P.M. Getting adequate sleep will help calm your overactive adrenals.

·························

Endocrine Disruptor: **TOO MUCH ALCOHOL**

It's Saturday night out with the girls, and by the bottom of the fourth bottle of Chianti at dinner you're flying out the door to the nearest dance floor, where you suck down vodka sodas throughout the night.

Managing the equation. Keep your pathways of elimination, especially the liver, open. Rehydrate and rebalance your blood sugar levels, which soared while boozing and then crashed—contributing to your awful hangover the next morning.

Food: Take a dose of inositol (a nutrient that helps detoxify the liver), vitamin C ester (a powerful antioxidant to combat the stress to your cells), as well as a B-vitamin complex (to recover more quickly from dehydration) before bed and when you wake up the next morning to help the liver detoxify. In addition, combine a serving of an electrolyte enhancer (I prefer Electro-Mix (by the makers of Emergen-C) with a tall glass of water and down it before you go to sleep. Consume three 8-ounce glasses of this detoxifying and rehydrating fresh juice throughout the next day (before breakfast, before lunch, and midafternoon). For each serving, combine a handful of spinach, 4 stalks of celery, half a cucumber, half a bunch of cilantro, one-third bunch of parsley, half a lemon with the rind, half a green apple, and a small carrot in a blender or juicer.

Exercise. Take a hatha yoga class (nothing heated or too intense). This will calm your adrenals, which are dealing with a lot of internal stress. The twists involved in yoga also help detoxify your internal organs to prevent a backup of estrogen.

Lifestyle. When you wake up the morning after drinking, make a commitment to start fresh that day. Oftentimes, drinking too much leads to eating too much for breakfast and then spending the rest of the day on the couch. Committing to a fresh start will prevent one unhealthy behavior from leading to another and will minimize any hormonal disruption that may occur from the excess alcohol.

....

Endocrine Disruptor: LATE-NIGHT CARB OVERLOAD

While cooking a delicious pasta dinner for you and your hubby, you work your way through a wedge of Gruyère; then, when the pasta is ready, you help yourself to a heaping bowl of penne with a slice of fresh rosemary-olive bread; finally, you munch on popcorn while working through the DVR queue.

Managing the equation. Immediately burn the glucose for fuel, prevent dehydration (due to excess carb intake) while you're sleeping, and increase the transit time through your system.

Food. Swallow 16 ounces of water before bed. Take a probiotic before bed to prevent the overgrowth of candida (yeast) in your gut from all the carbs. The next morning eat a protein-rich breakfast (such as an omelet or protein smoothie). Avoid both refined and complex carbohydrates the next day, except root vegetables (such as a sweet potato) and fruit.

Exercise. As soon as you notice that you've overindulged, climb the stairs in your home or go for a walk so that your muscles can help gobble up the glucose in your bloodstream.

Lifestyle. Discuss with your sweetheart other pleasurable activities you could do together besides overeating and sitting on the couch. For instance, take ballroom dancing lessons, go for hikes, learn to play tennis, or take cooking classes to learn how to make healthy meals together. Many couples fall into a routine of spending most of their quality time together relaxing, when you have so much more to gain (from both a health and a relationship standpoint) by choosing activities that keep you on your feet.

. . . .

✚ Your Yearly WomanCode Survival Kit

Reframe Your Mind-Set *Before* These Year-Round Events

. . . .

Event: VACATION

You've been looking forward to your Cabo vacation for months now, and the day has finally arrived. You head to the airport well before dawn and grab a blueberry muffin and large coffee to get yourself going. You pick up a salad to eat on the plane, but an hour into your flight you're so hungry that you scarf the free cookies, peanuts, and pretzels, too. You land at the airport and feel the warm sunshine on your skin. You check in to your hotel, change into your bathing suit, and head out to lunch with your girlfriends before spending the rest of the day at the beach. At dinner, you celebrate your first day in Mexico with an icy margarita, along with chicken enchiladas and an endless bowl of tortilla chips. The next four days consist of a pretty standard routine: waking up around noon, spending the day lying on the beach sipping cold beers, downing as much chips and salsa as you possibly can, and staying out late into the night drinking and dancing. You're on vacation, after all, and want to soak up every last moment of freedom before returning to reality at the end of the week.

Reframe your thinking. Most people use vacation as a time to ditch restraint and overindulge from the moment they pass through airport security until they return home. However, studies show that vacations just happen to be the best time to make lasting changes in your life. The reason: when you're in an unfamiliar environment, your brain is primed for forming the neural pathways that are associated with imprinting new behaviors. As you go about your everyday life at home, your brain functions on autopilot nearly all the time. (This explains why you're able to multitask a dozen different activities at once—you barely have to think!) And since autopilot is your default setting, your brain may find it difficult to learn new tricks. However, when you're on vacation, your brain is constantly being flooded with new experiences and new surroundings, and it adapts to them by forming new neural pathways.

You can take advantage of this process by deliberately throwing new behaviors into the mix. Your brain will be more likely to create the neural pathways necessary for making those behaviors automatic for you so that you can perform them with minimal effort once you return home. So as you prepare for your vacation, start thinking about how you could incorporate more of the WomanCode principles into your life while you're away. Perhaps it will be a time for you to fully try on the WomanCode lifestyle; alternatively, you could choose two or three activities that you might struggle with at home—such as moving your body daily or consuming mostly whole foods—and focus on making those activities new lifelong habits while you're away.

....

Event: BUSY TIME AT WORK

Work is as busy as it has ever been. You're buried under a pile of deadlines, juggling multiple projects, and gunning for a promotion. You're consistently clocking fourteen-hour days, including weekends, and can't remember the last time you caught more than six hours of shut-eye in a single night. (And when you're lucky enough to fall asleep, you awaken several times at night thinking about yet another item you have to accomplish the next day.) Those times when you actually remember to eat, your diet consists of venti peppermint mochas and any source of sugar you can find in the office pantry and vending machine. You and your coworkers have dinner delivered to the office each night—a daily rotation of pizza, Chinese, and burgers. The most physical activity you rack up during the day is trips to refill your coffee mug and the subsequent hikes to the bathroom when you can't hold it any longer. You're stressed, exhausted, and short-tempered, but see no signs of the intensity letting up if you're going to get noticed and score that coveted promotion.

Reframe your thinking. "I just need to get through this busy couple of weeks and then I'll get back to my normal healthy habits." Sound familiar? If so, I encourage you to ask yourself whether you ever truly get through those busy times. Isn't the reality of being a hardworking woman today the fact that you're perpetually busy? That there always seems to be more to do than you can actually get done? The longer you put off getting back to your normal healthy habits, the further away you'll ultimately find yourself from the state of health that you'd like to be in.

I'd like you to think about revising your mind-set and trying this on for size: "In order for me to function at the high level I expect of myself, I have to keep my body and mind in a peak state of health." For you to successfully take on everything that you want to accomplish, you need to be sleeping soundly, eating well, and moving your body so that your brain can be as productive and efficient as possible. The more work, stress, and obligations that pile up, the more you need to meet those challenges with extreme self-care. It's completely counterintuitive to what you may be used to doing, yet it makes perfect sense. You'd never expect an Olympic athlete to show up at an event without eating and training in a way that allows her to perform at her peak. The difference, of course, is that instead of competing every four years, every *day* may be an Olympic event for you. So you need to prime your body and mind for a gold-medal-caliber performance.

Here's how: prioritize your self-care routine as much as you do all the other responsibilities in your life. Just as you would a meeting at work or a call with a client, plug self-care tasks into your schedule as nonnegotiable items. Yes, put that ballet barre class on Tuesday nights into your planner. Pen in time to pick up groceries and prepare your meals for the week. If it helps to schedule sex, self-pleasure, or consistent bedtimes, then by all means write those in, too. Not only will maintaining regular self-care routines improve your focus and performance at work; they'll help you become more efficient. Remember that experiment from eighth-grade chemistry class where a gas expanded to fill any container, whether the volume of a water bottle or that of a shipping container? Well, work is the same exact way: it will always fill the amount of time that you give it. So giving yourself a clear cutoff time each day for you to incorporate these self-care activities means that you'll optimize the time that you spend working in order to leave ample space for your daily self-care to-dos.

....

***Event:* DRINKING TOO MUCH AND COPING WITH A HANGOVER**

It's your best friend's birthday party, and after a crazy few weeks with work you're relieved to have an opportunity to see your friends, celebrate, forget about everything, and let yourself go. You split several pitchers of sangria with your friends at the tapas dinner, and then spend the rest of the night in a booze-soaked blur, barhopping through town sucking down drink after drink. Somewhere around 3 A.M. you find yourself in a diner helping yourself to whatever's on the table—alternating between bites of cheese fries, buttermilk pancakes, and crispy fried chicken. Around dawn a cab delivers you to your apartment, where you dissolve onto your bed, fully clothed, and finally pass out.

Reframe your thinking. Well before you were twenty-one, you started to believe that the only way you could truly celebrate or let go was through inebriation of various sorts—alcohol, too many slices of chocolate cake, or drugs. But it doesn't have to be that way. Once you start to have a new, positive relationship with your body and you feel good all the time, it becomes clear that *you're* the only one who can make yourself feel happy. With that realization, you become less willing to compromise your well-being. However, you still want to spend time with your friends, and these situations often revolve around booze and greasy foods. Of course, spending quality time with your friends is just as crucial to your well-being as your other healthy habits. So how can you do this without sabotaging all your hard work?

It boils down to shifting your mind-set from using celebrations as an excuse to escape your body to using them to reach an even greater state of health, as well as forming even stronger relationships with the people in your life. The way I see it, you've worked hard to create a beautiful home for yourself in your body—why would you want to escape it anyway? For me, celebration is about having the time to spend with friends and loved ones, talking to them, and enjoying those moments. You can do that with a glass of club soda in your hand! You're also more present to the exchanges that you have when you're sober, which makes those connections much more powerful and fulfilling than waking up the next day and not being able to remember who was there. Even times when you're at a bar can be part of your self-care routine—taking the time to connect, touch, and dance your heart out when your favorite song is on. There's something about giving yourself over to the true joys in life with a completely clear head that makes you feel fully alive and is truly rewarding. And the best part is that you're even healthier because of it, instead of pouring health-hampering chemicals into your body.

I understand that sometimes it just feels like too much to skip alcohol altogether. In those instances when you have a drink or two, always stick to these guidelines:

- Limit your intake to no more than two drinks in a day.

- Choose alcohol with a lower glycemic load—sake, champagne, red wine and then white wine are your best choices. Avoid hard alcohol, mixed drinks, and beer.

- Follow each glass of alcohol with an 8-ounce glass of water.

- Never drink on an empty stomach. Always consume alcohol with food, which helps slow down the glucose uptake to your brain and liver. Choose something that has a little fat in it (though nothing fried), which will slow the glucose uptake even more. In terms of bar foods, my top recommendations are guacamole, nuts, or sushi.

•••••••••••••••••••••••••••••

Event: HOLIDAYS AND OTHER FAMILY TIMES

It's the holidays, which means you're on an endless circuit of parties and family gatherings from Halloween through New Year's Day. It's nearly impossible to resist all the treats that come out only this time of year, from the candy and fresh-baked pies to trays of decorated sugar cookies to the eggnog and festive canapés. When you head home to see your family, there's a constant parade of food from the moment you walk in the door. When your mom's not pushing her raspberry-ricotta French toast on you, it's your grandma shoving another slice of her homemade lasagna onto your plate, your aunt adding a scoop of vanilla ice cream to a slice of pecan pie, or your dad refilling your empty wine glass. You spend the holidays in a food coma, watching movies and football with your siblings during the day and catching up with high school friends in your favorite hometown bar at night.

Reframe your thinking. Many people use the winter holidays as an excuse to engage in poor self-care choices for about two months straight. There's also the complicated family dynamic that factors into these times—the fact that when we're breaking bread with loved ones, that shared activity builds community, loyalty, and trust. People show their love in many different ways, and for some it's through food. So you may fear that by not eating the food your family prepares, you may seem to be rejecting their love. You could even fear a sense of loneliness if you're not sharing the exact same food experience that everyone around you is.

But the crucial thing to realize when it comes to your family is that, above all, they truly want you to be happy and healthy. And in order to come from a place of love and joy during those times that you spend together, you need to take care of yourself physically and mentally. So I want you to imagine how different those occasions would be if you showed up the WomanCode way—feeling luminous and positive instead of stressed out and sick. You might be surprised at how well your family would accept the changes that you need to make in order to maintain this beautiful new state of being.

It's important that you stay true to those things that will keep you feeling well during this busy time. There's no question that you'll be faced with temptations during the holidays just about anywhere you go. It sounds a little odd, but to help keep yourself on track during the holidays (or any time of year, for that matter), try adopting the mind-set of a pregnant woman. A woman who's pregnant has no problem avoiding alcohol or other things that are harmful to her because she knows that they're not good for the baby either. Whether pregnant or not, *all* women should feel that same protective, maternal, self-prioritizing energy when it comes to their hormones. So think about which things will nourish your hormones and which will harm them.

When I first starting living this lifestyle fifteen years ago, I realized that I had to abandon basically all the staple foods of my family's diet—including pasta and bread—if I was going to get healthy. At first, that choice made me feel disconnected from my family, and it upset quite a few people because they felt like I was rejecting their way of life and their love. However, I've learned through this journey that as long as you're not trying to make other people change their habits (unless they ask directly for your guidance) and your interactions are free of judgment, your friends and relatives will come around and eventually feel less threatened by your personal changes. What's more, if you've taken charge of your endocrine system, you have the opportunity to lift everyone else higher during these celebrations, too, simply by sharing your positive energy.

Here are some practical tips that can help you get through the holidays and fully embrace the times that you spend with those closest to you:

- *Enjoy the holiday spread.* There will almost always be foods available that you can eat; you just need to know what they are. Look for the least processed items: salads, veggies, proteins, and whole grains are your smartest picks.

- **Offer to bring something to the holiday table.** One of the best ways to manage your carb intake at the holidays is to make a side dish that everyone can share, such as a wheatberry salad or wild rice pilaf.

- **Stock up on sweet potatoes.** They're a great option that you can roast or steam for a fiber-filled snack *before* heading to an event where you know there will be only a few healthy options available. If you're home for the holidays, you can also supplement what you can eat from the holiday spread with a sweet potato to create a more filling meal.

Staying Sensitive

As I noted earlier, another component of achieving a health-coach level of mastery is becoming more sensitive to your endocrine system's signals. You've already learned that the dynamic equation teaches you to listen to your endocrine system's cues and make adjustments as necessary. But what I didn't tell you is that these signals actually become easier to read over time.

I've been living this lifestyle for fifteen years, and I know that I can handle only a bite of a decadent dessert, such as flourless chocolate cake, without feeling the effects. Although my body may be better able to handle the sugar than it was fifteen years ago, when my blood sugar and hormones were still out of whack, my relationship with my body is so much deeper now that I feel the physical effects much sooner and more acutely. I'm so aware of the difference between feeling great and feeling terrible that going any further in an unhealthy direction isn't worth it for me. This is what I mean by becoming more sensitive.

Sensitivity requires a dramatic shift from how you may have felt in the past, when you were very *desensitized* to your body's signals. We're often so busy that we forget to connect the dots between what we eat and what we feel. (If you've ever overeaten when you were already stuffed, you know exactly what I mean.) But this is true, too, when it comes to symptoms such as bloating, fatigue, constipation, headaches, or mood swings *even if you eat an appropriate amount* of a certain food that simply doesn't agree with your body and your hormones. This disconnect makes it extremely difficult to trace your symptoms back to what you did or what you ate; in fact, you may not even realize that your symptoms and your food intake are related. But now you know they are. You were also desensitized to the connection between the foods you eat and your reproductive health, so it was impossible to tie something you put in your body to a symptom you experienced in return.

So how does a person become more sensitive? Self-awareness is 90 percent of the battle. At this point in your journey, you've got that part licked: you've already been doing steps 1 through 4 of the protocol for weeks or months now. When you put something into your system that's not on the protocol, you notice it. Even if you don't pay attention intensely, you still feel the effects immediately. These effects may be similar to what you experienced before; but now, armed with knowledge about how your endocrine system works and your newfound mind-set of partnering with your body, these effects become impossible to ignore. You've also cleaned up your body in such a profound way that you've made your endocrine system much more efficient, which in turn makes you more sensitive. Not only do you notice the symptoms the endocrine disruptor has created; you're now in a position, with the knowledge you gained in this chapter, to counterbalance the effects and prevent that disruption from happening to you again.

I understand if you're thinking: "Why would I want these things to make me feel even *worse*?" To this I say: the thing to fear isn't becoming more sensitive; rather, it's not having the ability to sense what your body is desperately trying to tell you or ignoring your body when it sends you those signals that is scary. Doing so can take you far in the wrong direction. That's when you become the most vulnerable to hormonal breakdown. And we can all agree that you don't want to go there ever again. But when you're not aware, not listening, and not responding to your endocrine system's signals, bad behaviors can have a snowball effect. Sensitivity allows you to prevent all of that from happening: you can stop yourself the moment you notice that you've taken a step in a potentially damaging direc-

Cutting Out Wheat and Dairy

Most women suffering from any of the three categories of hormonal conditions—menstrual, fertility, or libido—can benefit greatly from removing dairy and wheat (specifically, gluten) from their diet. There are several reasons why:

- *Dairy is a loaded with estrogen. It contains 60 to 80 percent of the estrogen consumed in the American diet. What's more, cows on most modern dairy farms are pregnant nearly year-round, and milk from a knocked-up cow contains about 33 percent more of a certain kind of estrogen that can affect the human body than milk from cows that aren't pregnant. While the last thing any woman with a hormone-driven condition needs is adding more estrogen into the mix, this is especially true for women dealing with fibroids and endometriosis. Estrogen has growth-stimulating effects in your body (just as it causes us to grow and mature in puberty), and these can make the excess tissue growth you're already experiencing with fibroids and endometriosis even worse.*

- *Casein (the indigestible portion of dairy) and gluten (the indigestible portion of wheat) elicit an inflammatory response in the small intestine,*

tion. Then you can put all the skills you learned in this chapter to work as you clean up any damage that was done and get back to a state of endocrine equilibrium.

There's more good news: you won't be über-sensitive forever. The longer you follow the WomanCode protocol, the more your endocrine system will be operating under ideal circumstances. For those times when you fall off the protocol, you'll still feel sensitive to the effects, but you'll bounce back much more quickly than you did at the start. You'll also have much more experience with the tools in this chapter that help you get back on track, meaning that you can seamlessly call them into action for an even quicker return to health.

whether or not you're allergic to them. Although you can have occasional doses of these things and the body neutralizes the inflammatory response with antioxidants from the diet, the reality is that all of us are overexposed, so our small intestine is constantly in an inflamed state. This compromises your ability to properly absorb all the nutrients from the foods that you eat.

• Both dairy and wheat tend to slow transit time through the large intestine. This increases estrogen dominance, because your body can't clear that hormone out of your system quickly enough. When you're not going to the bathroom regularly, estrogen permeates the lining of the large intestine and makes its way back into your bloodstream, leading to an excess of estrogen in your body.

Because a major part of living in partnership with your body is learning how it reacts to the foods you eat, I encourage you to experiment with your own degree of dairy and gluten sensitivity. Instead of solely trusting my word, recognizing and understanding your individual reactions to these foods will make it much easier for you to make decisions at every meal. You'll know from experience how they make **you** feel. To assess your dairy and gluten sensitivity, try the two six-day sensitivity tests.

One-on-One with Alisa

In this chapter, I've given you a new way of looking at those things that can send you off track on your WomanCode journey. I've helped you see that instead of falling off the wagon, self-punishing, and digging yourself into a deeper hole, you have the power to change your body and make yourself feel better right away. To reinforce just how dynamic

· ·

Are You Sensitive to Dairy?

- *For two consecutive days, eat dairy with three meals each day, such as milk with cereal at breakfast, yogurt with lunch, and cheese with dinner.*

- *For the next two consecutive days, remove all dairy from your diet. Read package labels to make sure you're not accidentally consuming it.*

- *On the next day, have a dairy-free breakfast and lunch. Then, in the middle of the afternoon, around 3:30 or 4 p.m., eat a good-size serving of dairy on an empty stomach. Twenty minutes after eating, tune in to any stomach symptoms. Do you have any pain or belching? Do you have any nasal congestion or a runny nose? Do you have a headache? Is there a rash or hives on your skin? Evaluate your symptoms two hours later, again looking for any bloating, gassiness, or flatulence.*

- *Finally, the next morning, notice whether your bowels were affected. Are they loose? Are you constipated?*

If you have any of the symptoms listed above, you're very likely sensitive to dairy. Taking a few months off all dairy can do wonders for your body and increase your success while following the WomanCode protocol. You can then decide whether you'd like to gradually add dairy back in or stay on a dairy-free diet for the long term. With so many calcium-rich dairy alternatives, this is much easier than ever. If you restore dairy to your diet and notice any returning symptoms, I strongly urge you to remove it for the long-term.

this power is, and to reinforce the value of making those good choices, I'd love for you to get very clear about what happens when you get off—and right back on—course. Try these activities to gain that clarity:

- Write about a recent time when you got out of your FLO. What was the situation? Did you go out drinking with your coworkers on Friday night? Did you have a few too many sweets last weekend? Describe the experience.

Are You Sensitive to Gluten?

- For two consecutive days, eat wheat-based products with three meals, such as cereal for breakfast, a sandwich for lunch, and pasta for dinner.
- For two consecutive days, remove all gluten-containing products from your diet. Read labels to make sure everything you eat is gluten-free.
- The next day, eat a gluten-free diet until dinner. Then, at dinner, have a substantial amount of a gluten-containing food, such as pizza or pasta. Twenty minutes after eating, tune in to any symptoms. Do you have any pain or belching? Is there any swelling in your lower abdomen? Do you have any nasal congestion or a runny nose? Do you have a headache? Is there a rash or hives on your skin? Evaluate your symptoms two hours later, again looking for any bloating, gassiness, or flatulence.
- Finally, the next morning, notice whether your bowels were affected. Are you constipated?

If you notice any of the symptoms listed above, you are gluten-sensitive. Though you may not have celiac disease, you can still be sensitive enough to gluten to have it be an obstacle for your digestive health and overall well-being. Remove gluten from your diet for several months and notice what kind of difference it makes. If the difference is significant, you may choose to keep gluten out for the long term. If you decide to add it back in and experience renewed symptoms, I encourage you to stay on a gluten-free diet to protect your endocrine system's health.

- Then, what changes did you make to get back on track? If you'd had too much to drink, did you down some B vitamins and electrolytes when you got home? Did you eat well the next day? Write down exactly what you did that helped.

- What positive changes did you observe in your body? For example, did you prevent a hangover? If you ate a sugar-rich meal and followed it with a protein-rich meal, did you avoid a bellyache and blood sugar crash? When you put these tools into action, what are the effects you feel in the body and how different are those effects from what you're used to experiencing?

- Share the experience with someone you know and with us on Facebook. This is one of the best ways to ensure that you'll make these wise choices again in the future. That's because you can clearly see how amazing you are, how incredible your body is, and how you and your body are creating a beautiful new relationship *working together* toward a more pleasurable experience in your skin.

Finally, it's time to do a little planning. Look at the week ahead and plan what you can do to stay on your WomanCode journey and in your FLO:

- Chart out the next week. What events or occasions may make you vulnerable to being knocked off track? Do you have any family gatherings planned? A birthday party for a friend? An upcoming vacation? A stressful time at work?

- Using the tools I've already given you, along with your own creativity, for each occasion write down what your new plan of action will be.

Practice this skill at the start of every week as a way to always put your hormonal health first.

SUCCESS STORY: Heidi Braun, 40

CONDITION: Ovarian Cysts

My healing journey began in February at my annual ob-gyn exam. A routine sonogram to check a fibroid revealed that I had developed cysts—one on each ovary—measuring two centimeters. I didn't want surgery! When I asked my doctor about proactive steps, her only advice was to monitor them and she would see me in two months for another sonogram. What?! Not being one to just sit around for two months and do the whole "wait and see" thing, I started the WomanCode program.

My initial sessions with Alisa focused on my lifestyle—diet, activities, relationships—it was all about the positive and working together. She put me on supplements to help my body process hormones better. I started drinking more water. That was coupled with food experiments—what healthy foods satisfied and sustained me. My whole diet changed.

A month into my program, I felt better . . . lighter . . . both physically and emotionally.

In the third month it was time to go back for another sonogram. Alisa and I spoke prior to my visit and she told me not to expect any changes. I was fine with that. I knew I was doing all I could and they were great things for my health nonetheless. So as I lay on the table, with no expectations, the technician tells me, "The cyst on the left ovary is gone" and then "Oh! The one on the right is gone, too!" I'm in shock. I'm elated. And as a tear rolls down my cheek, I'm in awe of the power . . . the power this body has to heal itself. How amazing is that! If I treat it right (if I treat me right), then amazing things will happen.

Ladies, change is never easy. It's not an all or nothing process. By putting certain changes into action, you will see firsthand what your awesome, powerful, strong bodies can do. This was and will continue to be a life-changing event in my life. And can you believe all these good things started with two cysts?

PART III

BECOMING A POWER SOURCE

CHAPTER 7

Optimize Your Fertility

O nce upon a time, to get pregnant women and men had sex. It was generally easy, enjoyable, and free. Today, that's not always the case. One in eight couples confronts fertility issues. One in one hundred babies is conceived in a test tube. In this day and age, fertility is something that we, as women, need to be actively engaged in protecting and preserving. Everything in our environment, including what we put on and into our bodies, has the potential to disrupt our fertility.

Several years ago a woman came to my center because she was having trouble getting pregnant. She was a trader working on the floor of the New York Stock Exchange, handling hundred-million-dollar deals on a daily basis. She was brilliant, completely stressed out, her cycles were unpredictable, she barely slept, and she was getting by on coffee, salads, and sandwiches. Yet she was in total disbelief that she hadn't been able to conceive.

I see this all the time. As women, we expect that getting pregnant is something we should be able to do. We put so much energy into trying *not* to get pregnant for so long that we believe conception will happen quickly and effortlessly when we decide that the time is right. And it *should* be easy—except for the fact that we live in a complicated world where we believe getting ahead comes at the expense of our bodies. We live in a toxic environment that's robbing us of our birthright to have healthy cycles, healthy fertility, and abundant energy and libido throughout our lives.

But there's great news: living in the FLO will safeguard your fertility. Regardless of whether or not you're trying to conceive at this moment in your life, making these diet and lifestyle changes will ensure that your fertility will be there for you when you want it. First and foremost, the WomanCode protocol ensures that estrogen is eliminated from your body properly. This is crucial, because elevated levels of estrogen can confuse the brain-ovary conversation. If you have too much estrogen piled up in your bloodstream, a variety of scenarios can take place, from overgrowth of endometrium, development of cysts or fibroids, to premature ovarian failure and thus an inability to become pregnant. Yet you can literally improve your fertility by living in the FLO of your hormones and following the WomanCode protocol, making sure that your body is properly metabolizing and excreting estrogen through your pathways of elimination. The WomanCode lifestyle also supports your overall endocrine and ovarian function to preserve your fertility. It does this in part by encouraging a diet rich in fruits and vegetables that nourish your ovaries and eggs with antioxidants, including glutathione, which is essential for healthy egg quality. (There will be more on the importance of smart food choices for fertility in a moment.) With more women today wanting to give birth later in life than ever before (and more power to us for that!), it's even more crucial that we do everything we can to protect our reproductive organs so that they'll be there for us when we need them most.

Whether you're still years away from finding Mr. Right, are actively trying to conceive, are in your third cycle of IVF, or are in the early stages of perimenopause and wanting to get pregnant, this chapter is for you. I want to help you appreciate the ability that you have to preserve and enhance your own fertility. It sounds like a lot of responsibility—and it is—but it's also incredibly empowering. In addition to knowing which foods are important to use on top of the WomanCode protocol for fertility, women I work with are frequently surprised to learn just how powerful the shifting of certain habits or beliefs about their bodies can be when it comes to getting pregnant. This is true whether you want to get pregnant later this year or later this decade.

Your body is designed to conceive and stay pregnant. Your endocrine system—a.k.a. your WomanCode—is there to do all the heavy lifting. All I want you to do is to clear a path for it to keep your body hormonally primed for easy conception and successful pregnancy. Eating the WomanCode way, detoxifying your home, choosing organic and free-range foods, and increasing outlets for creativity, pleasure, and rest should be your exclusive focus. Getting pregnant in our modern world can often be an emotional and stressful process. I have found that the stress experienced by my clients is greatly reduced when they take action. They want to know all the possible ways that they can be proactively improving their internal fertility environment. I want to share with you these additional WomanCode key ways to dramatically improve your fertility.

- *Improve Rates of Successful Implantation/Conception.*
  I mentioned earlier a study that concluded that your period is an indicator of overall health. That menstrual-related hormonal imbalances, if left untreated, lead to diseases of inflammation. Inflammation has been well-established as an obstacle to successful conception, whether by natural means or by IVF methods. We've seen how foods can reduce inflammation and increase hormonal balance. I cannot stress enough how critical it is for you to get started on having the best periods possible

now for your long-term fertility protection and your short-term conception success. These are ways for you to see what your body is trying to tell you about your ability to conceive. If you are noticing any of these cycle symptoms, make sure you are following the WomanCode protocol immediately.

- **Ensure you can maintain the pregnancy.** Observing the luteal phase of your cycle is key for you to most easily understand how prepared your progesterone levels are to sustain a pregnancy in those critical first few weeks. First, look specifically at the length of the phase—is it shorter than ten days or longer than twelve to fourteen days? If so, progesterone levels will likely be too low for pregnancy, though you may successfully conceive. You can work with your doctor to avoid miscarriages if you are able to bring this information forward. Second, document the intensity of your PMS symptoms—how many are there and how severe are they? Acne, headaches, insomnia, breast tenderness, cystic breasts, bloating, and mood swings all indicate a disproportionate ratio of estrogen to progesterone. This balance must be optimal for you to keep the pregnancy. In addition, consult "Seeing Red" on page 154 to help further identify ways in which your actual menstruation week is telling you about your hormonal balance.

- **Identify hidden fertility obstacles.** Look beyond your cycle to see what else your body is trying to tell you about your hormonal well-being, your levels of inflammation, and your nutrient availability, all of which impact successful conception, pregnancy, and egg quality. How are your bowel movements? Remember that chronic mild constipation can exacerbate estrogen dominance, while IBS with diarrhea can lead to small intestine inflammation that blocks key nutrient absorption.

All those supplements you are taking to boost your folic acid levels, for example, won't have as much of an impact if your digestive and elimination systems are flowing smoothly and calmly. Do a body scan of your skin for acne, eczema, rosacea, rashes, or other types of irritation. Your skin has a deep connection to your liver and will show you how well the liver is doing. Skin inflammation means liver congestion and congestion will lead to compromised ability to metabolize estrogen and that will throw off that ideal hormonal ratio for baby. What's your emotional temperature? If you're struggling with anxiety, depression, irritability, and/or insomnia, these all indicate lower levels of vitamin D3 and omega-3 fatty acids, both key nutrients in utilizing and stabilizing hormone levels and can be linked to low progesterone levels as well.

- **_Get a clean bill of sexual health._** Finally, do what you can to create a sperm- and embryo-friendly internal environment. Chronic bacterial overgrowth and STDs have been linked to decreased fertility rates. Address chronic BV (bacterial vaginosis), UTIs (urinary tract infections), and yeast infections—all of which disturb your delicate vaginal pH balance and when disrupted make the journey for the sperm to the egg much more difficult. In addition, get checked for HPV and chlamydia—two extremely common STDs that can create a less than optimal environment for the embryo.

Remember that by doing the WomanCode protocol, you will be eating to optimize your weekly hormonal ratios. When trying to conceive, pay extra attention to this, making sure you are:

- incorporating sprouted and fermented foods during the follicular phase to deliver as many bioavailable nutrients as possible to the ovary

- consuming the majority of your fruits and vegetables raw during ovulation to up egg-boosting glutathione levels

- eating liver-supportive sweet root vegetables, like sweet potatoes, and leafy greens from the brassica family, like kale, during the luteal phase to make sure you are eliminating estrogen efficiently and keeping an optimal ration of estrogen and progesterone for pregnancy maintenance

- replenish your minerals during your menstrual phase by consuming sea vegetables, avocados, and/or some free-range animal protein to deeply nourish your endocrine system for the next cycle

Developing a more intimate relationship with your ovaries and uterus is also a way to reduce the stress and anxiety so common with the uncertainty of this process. Visualize them glowing, healthy, and happy while you meditate on the fact that you are a fertile vessel, designed to receive and create. If you can put your attention on dramatically improving your self-care and turning your nurturing energy on to managing your hormonal health, then you will not only be practicing the very skills you'll need as a mother, but you'll also enjoy this journey of pregnancy much more.

Creating Space for a Baby

Women who come to me with fertility problems often fall into one of three camps. There are women like the adrenal-fried trader who've been burning the candle at both ends throughout their adult lives. Then there are women such as the nurses and teachers I work with who have dedicated their entire lives to helping others and have left little for themselves. Finally, there are women who've recently gone off the Pill, many having been on it since they were teenagers, and discovered that the synthetic hormones had been masking an underlying functional issue that's now blocking their ability to conceive. All of these women share an important commonality, and you may, too: they haven't been living in partnership with their bodies.

As an endocrine-focused health coach, it's my privilege to help women move back into their bodies, as it were. Helping to repair that partnership is the most crucial step in helping women overcome fertility issues and get pregnant. Once *you* begin living in partnership with *your* body, it will be there for you to use however you like—conceiving and maintaining a healthy pregnancy is no exception.

I want you to think about each phase of your cycle as an opportunity to take proper nutritional care of your code, to cross-train your life, and reprioritize for baby. I'm going to ask you a question that probably no ob-gyn would ever bring up: What are you willing to shift in your life in order to be an ideal vessel for conception? It's not something many of us talk about, because we assume that having a pair of fully functioning ovaries should be enough. But as any woman who has struggled with fertility can attest, conceiving is often more complicated than the clinical detail of a sperm meeting an egg. It's an emotional experience that requires so much more than a roll in the hay to happen.

From an energetic standpoint, pregnancy may be eluding you because there isn't enough space in your life for that pregnancy or, more importantly, for the baby who would be dependent on you for every life-sustaining need nine months from now. From a physical standpoint, shifting your life to make space for a pregnancy and a baby is crucial for conception because shifting your life means slowing down. And when you slow down, you send a signal to your endocrine system (the HPA axis, in particular) that there's no physical threat to your well-being and that your body is in prime condition for a developing fetus to thrive.

Learning to slow down begins by shifting your priorities and living your life as if you already had a child. One of the most common problems I see in women who have trouble conceiving is that they've overextended their lives. This leaves them feeling drained and stands in their way of being a viable vessel for a baby. Activities that make you feel overextended will ultimately seem insignificant and fall by the wayside once you're caring for a newborn. Don't wait to let them go. Put to use the cross-training tools you learned in chapter 5 and reprioritize. Try thinking about how you would live your life if you already had a baby. Of course, this doesn't mean giving up every Saturday night with your girlfriends and pretending you have an infant at home. Rather, it means saying no to commitments that push you over the limit of what you're able to accomplish without feeling completely burned out, so that your cortisol levels stay balanced and your adrenals stay healthy. It means setting boundaries so that, instead of giving everything you have to everyone else, you leave some energy for yourself to prepare and eat the foods you know you should to prevent hypoglycemia. It means building self-care (whether cooking a nutritious meal, going for a jog, or taking a relaxing bath) into your schedule and following through with it just as you would any other appointment. When new opportunities arise, ask yourself, *Will this activity charge my battery or drain it?* Try to minimize those that tax your energy, because they're also likely to tax your health and, ultimately, your fertility. Start looking at your life from a new perspective: examine how you could put an end to overextending in order to make space for a baby if you got pregnant tomorrow.

Fertility-Boosting Foods and Supplements

In traditional cultures, men and women were fed a premarital meal believed to optimize fertility so that they'd have a greater chance at conceiving on their wedding night. While this bygone approach may have missed the mark (one meal won't make a difference), our ancestors were headed in the right direction (*consistent* consumption of certain foods *will* enhance fertility). Modern science is catching up to this belief and has recently shown that choosing particular foods can, in fact, boost the health of a woman's reproductive system and increase her chances of conceiving and maintaining a healthy pregnancy. One recent study found that women store omega-3 fatty acids in the fat tissue of our hips and thighs that a fetus depends on while developing in utero. So long before you become pregnant, your diet is crucial for creating an optimal environment for a baby. Since your body can't manufacture omega-3s on its own, those nutrients have to come from the food that we eat. Another recent study found that curcumin, the active ingredient in the spice turmeric, is a powerful anti-inflammatory. Inflammation can compromise the genetic material of your eggs, so consuming turmeric in your diet can protect this genetic material, increase blood flow to the ovaries, thus keeping them healthier, and improve the chances of conceiving and of maintaining a healthy pregnancy.

Food choices are crucial not only for women trying to conceive naturally. Brand-new research has found that what a woman eats and drinks can also affect her success with infertility treatments such as IVF. In one Harvard study, researchers found that women having IVF who consumed the most saturated fats (primarily found in animal sources such as red meat) had fewer mature oocytes (cells that form eggs), which reduced their likelihood of successful infertility treatment. Meanwhile, women with the highest intake of monounsaturated fats (found in foods such as nuts, seeds, avocados, vegetable oils, and nut butters) were about three and a half times more likely to have a live birth than women who consumed the least. Another study, in Denmark, found that drinking more than five cups of coffee per day reduced women's chances of becoming pregnant with IVF

••

IVF and Egg Freezing

*IVF is a process that can be very stressful on the ovary and, as is well-documented, is not a guaranteed method of ensuring conception. While it can be hugely helpful for some women, more often than not, the cause of infertility for individual women has no known cause according to standard medicine. Your best insurance policy, whether you end up choosing this route or not needing it, is to feed your ovaries, and keep your hormones balanced using the WomanCode method. I've seen too many women come to my center after they have done three to five rounds of IVF and have put their relationships and bodies through the hormonal mood swing wringer, and now their ovaries have been hyper-stimulated and the doctor is recommending a significant break in treatment. It's important for you to consider the effects of this chemical manipulation of your ovaries on egg quality and reserve before you go through multiple rounds without taking on the essential nutritional support your body needs to have this experience be successful. Nutritional research is absolutely confirming that certain foods have a dramatic impact on the IVF process as well as promoting egg quality. As mentioned above, eating avocado (high in prized monounsaturated fat) while going through IVF has been proven to increase the chance of pregnancy 3.4 times versus those women who did not consume adequate amounts of this nutrient. Food works! It would make sense, then, that when you consult with a fertility specialist, that this information would be readily available to you. I have heard too many stories of women asking their doctors specifically about this and being told at most to avoid caffeine and alcohol, which is very good advice considering the studies listed above. Please don't be frustrated with your doctors, **ever**. They are all extremely* treatment by about 50 percent compared with women who didn't drink any coffee at all. This doesn't surprise me, since excess caffeine can alter blood sugar, overstimulate the adrenals, and affect elimination, all which disrupt your hormonal balance.

skilled technicians of the human body and, in the world of IVF specialists and reproductive endocrinologists, they can be enormous allies for you in your journey to conceive. Until, however, there is more research, and more functional nutrition taught in medical schools, it will always be the rare physician who readily offers this information to you. The healthcare system assumes the patient will be relatively passive in her treatment, both in the hospital setting and after, beyond taking medications. But I do see a future in which all women going through IVF are prescribed the WomanCode protocol by their doctors as their first course of action. **Just as you would want to feed yourself the best foods while pregnant, you want to be feeding your eggs and ovaries the most nutrient-dense foods before conception too.** A healthy baby is formed from nature and nurture—the nature of her DNA and the nurturing of maternal diet. If you are thinking about IVF or egg freezing and are worried about ovarian hyper-stimulation, it's important to consider how hormonally sensitive you are to begin with (how easy or difficult it was for you to find a pill that worked well for your body, for example), as that is an excellent indicator of how well you'll tolerate the injectable hormones.

Egg freezing is similar in many ways to the IVF process, the obvious omission being an immediate implantation. The data on egg viability after this process remains to be determined as more and more women use this option. Studies have shown that the younger you "bank your eggs," the better the viability (under the age of thirty being best). The reality, however, is that most women are not thinking about such things until they are closer to forty. So assuming you do go ahead with this process later on in your hormonal lifespan, it's even more essential for you to engage the WomanCode protocol, to keep your body primed for the moment you decide to implant and try for conception.

There's another key reason why what you eat matters for your fertility: stress. Earlier, you learned that it's helpful for conception that your hypothalamus and pituitary gland must receive the all-clear message from your adrenals that there's no threat to your well-being. However, if you're eating a nutrient-deprived diet, your adrenals register this as a form of internal stress, and this response can signal to the brain that this might not be an ideal time for pregnancy for you or baby. Here's how. When stress is high, your cortisol levels rise and production of the hormone DHEA—a hormone from which many other hormones, including progesterone and estrogen, are created—drops. In effect, then, internal stress prevents the optimal hormonal environment for conceiving and maintaining a pregnancy.

Your body requires a complex variety of nutrients to function optimally. When it's not getting enough of these nutrients or it's receiving too many harmful ones (such as saturated fats and refined carbohydrates), this is stressful for your body, as we just saw. On top of that, when your organs are dedicated to flushing these toxins from your system, they don't have the space or energy to work toward helping you become pregnant. The good news, however, is that while there are very few *external* stressors you can control (such as crazy deadlines and horrific bosses), you can limit *internal* stress by eating a high-quality diet (which in turn helps to mitigate the potential damage from external stress).

The diet and lifestyle protocol described in this book is designed to correct any physical blockages and underlying hormonal issues that could be keeping you from getting pregnant. In addition to those dietary and lifestyle changes, the following list of foods can have particular benefits for your fertility (including those rich in compounds such as omega-3 fatty acids, curcumin, and monounsaturated fats).

Top-Ten WomanCode Favorite Fertility-Boosting Foods

Fill your daily diet with these foods, which contain a variety of fertility-fueling nutrients:

- *Buckwheat.* This grain is rich in the compound d-chiro-inositol, which has been proven to drop insulin and testosterone levels and increase rates of ovulation, thereby improving fertility.

- *Leafy greens.* Spinach, kale, collards, and escarole, among many others, are high in folic acid, which is essential for healthy ovaries and reduces the risk of spinal cord or brain defects in infants. They are also rich in vitamin E, magnesium, and calcium, which promote menstrual cycle health.

- *Chickpeas.* Just one serving of this legume can maintain proper B6 levels, which are essential for the production of healthy progesterone levels for conception, as well as improving sperm and egg development.

- *Honey.* All honey, but especially bee pollen and royal jelly—the queen bee's favorite dish—is a nutrient-rich compound with many features. While being fed royal jelly by the worker bees, queen bees lay up to two thousand eggs each day. Bee pollen can help stimulate ovarian function when trying to conceive.

- *Eggs.* These ancient symbols of fertility sometimes get a bum rap. Don't skip the yolks! Free-range egg yolks contain vitamin D, which is essential in maintaining healthy ovulation.

- *Sunflower Seeds.* Rich in zinc—which helps your body more efficiently utilize your reproductive hormones (estrogen and progesterone) and also helps with DNA production that can support egg quality.

- **Salmon.** Omega-3 fatty acids, which salmon has in abundance, helps in regulating hormones and ovulation, while also increasing cervical mucus and blood flow to the reproductive organs.

- **Avocados.** They're high in monounsaturated fat, which has been shown to positively affect IVF outcomes.

- **Cinnamon.** In addition to its antibacterial and digestion-improving properties, cinnamon contains a compound that makes fat cells more responsive to insulin, which in turn increases ovulation rates.

- **Turmeric.** Not only will this spice boost the health of your reproductive system; it—along with other similar "warming" spices, such as coriander, cumin, cardamom, and black pepper—helps dispel, according to TCM (traditional Chinese medicine), excessive dampness in the reproductive organs. It helps create a drier, warmer internal environment that's ideal for conception.

Hormone-Enhancing Supplements

The next time you visit your ob-gyn, ask her to perform a blood panel to obtain readings on key levels of certain hormones: progesterone, estrogen, follicle-stimulating hormone (FSH), and luteinizing hormone (LH). She will then interpret that information to help you understand where your levels are. (If you've been struggling with conceiving for some time, you may already know where you stand.) Once you have that information, use the chart below to find the appropriate supplements that will work with your body to support hormonal balance in the short term. You can try these supplements for one to three months.

If estrogen is low	If progesterone is low	If FSH or LH is abnormal
Take dong quai.	*Use wild yam cream from ovulation to day 28 of your menstrual cycle on areas of your body where skin is thinnest, such as your elbows and behind your knees, as well as on your lower belly.*	*Take vitex daily.*
This product, a member of the parsley family, made from the roots of this plant, will help balance estrogen levels that support the tissue lining the uterus. This tissue, which is often inadequate when estrogen is low, is necessary for housing the embryo.	*It naturally boosts progesterone levels to help the uterine lining stay in place for successful conception.*	*Extracted from the fruit and seeds of the chasteberry tree, this herbal supplement improves pituitary gland secretion of FSH and LH.*

For women trying to conceive. It's important to pay extra attention to your vaginal secretions during the four phases of your menstrual cycle. In the ovulation phase, you're looking for the fluid to be clear, with the consistency of uncooked egg white. If that's happening, it's a great sign for your fertility. The egg is perfectly positioned for implantation and conception during this phase, so have sex once a day for two to three consecutive days. Climaxing during intercourse floods your body with oxytocin and nitric oxide (read more about them in chapter 8) and thus improves your chances for conception.

Fertile Lives, Fertile Bodies

Beyond just making space and reorganizing priorities to decrease stress in your life (and the toll that stress takes on your HPA axis, ovulation, and hormone production), I also encourage you to cultivate a sense of being fertile in areas of your life besides your uterus. In other words, be creative!

You may not realize that, baby or no baby, you already give birth to things every single day. I deeply believe that as women, we're designed to be fertile in all areas of our lives. What's more, many of us create so often and so effortlessly that we miss the opportunity to acknowledge what we've created and to give ourselves permission to enjoy our creations. In 2007, the consulting firm McKinsey & Company published a study which found that those companies in which women are most strongly represented in top-management positions perform the best. In 2011, a study published in the *Harvard Business Review* reported that the collective intelligence of teams in

Can You Still Get Pregnant in Perimenopause?

In a word: yes. Women technically enter the first part of perimenopause between the ages of thirty-five and forty-four, but it's perfectly reasonable to consider conceiving naturally during this time. Although your levels of progesterone and estrogen start to decline, it's a very slow and gradual process, especially in the earlier years. The sooner you start living the WomanCode protocol, the slower this process will occur, because you're supporting these hormonal ratios in a very proactive way. Following the protocol also helps you feel calm about your fertility, since you know you're doing everything in your power to optimize it. (Trying to conceive can create a stressful experience for many women, as you may know from personal experience, and low stress levels are essential to help keep the adrenals—and thus hormone production—healthy.)

In addition to following the protocol, be sure to embrace the recommendations I've made in this chapter to support your fertility even further from a physical and energetic standpoint. It's especially important that you fill your diet with plenty of fertility-boosting foods to make sure your reproductive organs and hormones are in the best possible shape for conceiving and maintaining a healthy pregnancy.

the workplace rises when more female members are added. There is no doubt in my mind that both of these findings are due to women's innate ability to create. It's not just our ability to create new ideas and new opportunities that lifts everyone up, but also our ability to create within the context of our careers and our relationships.

Consciously identifying those things that you create and nurture in your life is a process that I call cultivating a fertile mind-set. It's about bringing your attention to what you birth, and recognizing those things as valuable and worthy of your energy, time, resources, and care. When you begin to look at (and respect) all those things

Here are some additional recommendations if you're in perimenopause and trying to become pregnant:

- *Have your doctor perform a comprehensive blood workup. It's important to identify any hormonal problems as soon as possible, to address them and give yourself ample time to conceive naturally.*

- *Seek out a uterine massage practitioner. This form of massage will improve blood flow and circulation to your reproductive organs as well as break up any physical adhesions that can interfere with implantation. Clear Passage is an excellent resource.*

- *Work with an acupuncturist and let him or her know that you're trying to conceive. A skilled practitioner will target the Ren channel—a meridian associated with conception in Chinese medicine.*

- *Break up the amount of time you spend sitting each day. If you're in your late thirties, you're likely in the full swing of your career and may spend a lot of time at your desk every day. This can deprive your uterus and reproductive organs of the blood flow and nourishment they need, so take a break from sitting every hour to stand up and walk around. This will help prevent any kind of stagnation in that area.*

that you create on a daily basis, you tap into your natural state of fertility/abundance and align your energy with the physical act of conception, pregnancy, and birth every day. By cultivating a fertile mind-set you up the ante: while you are working on improving the function of your endocrine system using the food piece of the protocol, you are also simultaneously bringing yourself into harmony with your birthright as a creative life force.

You don't need to out-craft Martha Stewart or decorate an apartment worthy of a spread in a magazine to feel like you've created something. The things you give birth to in your daily life may be far subtler. In a recent conversation on the phone with an old friend, I noticed that she was heading down a path of negativity. With just a few words I was able to take our conversation in a much more positive direction, so instead of feeling tired and drained after our talk, we both hung up the phone feeling energized and connected. I *created* that positive shift in our conversation and our relationship. Using the fertile mind-set, I took a moment to identify what I could create in that moment, and then took pleasure in acknowledging the difference it made for both of us.

To begin cultivating a fertile mind-set—which, by the way, I encourage you to do whether you're trying to get pregnant or not—give this exercise a try: ask yourself, *What do I already do in my life that I can identify as something I've created?* Perhaps you're great at creating opportunities, such as getting your girlfriends together for dinner once a month. Maybe you're especially good at creating delicious meals and sharing them with the people you love. As you go about your day, take note of the things that happen because you created them. You'll quickly realize that you are already in the vibration necessary for creating and sustaining a life and thus will become more aligned—emotionally and physically—to the possibility.

SUCCESS STORY: Katie Reimer, 32

CONDITION: Difficulty with Fertility

When I first went to the FLO Living Center in 2009, I had been taking the Pill for more than a decade. My doctor put me on it as a teenager because my menstrual cycles were three or four months apart. But I knew I wanted to have kids someday soon, and I didn't want to be on the Pill for the rest of my life. I didn't want something synthetic controlling my body. I just wanted to embrace what my body was giving me. And that's exactly what I discovered while working with the WomanCode program. The nutrition information was incredibly useful, and I continue to use it today. But the most important thing I gained was learning to work with my body. I came to understand that although my cycles were unique, that they were all mine.

Then, in 2010, my husband and I decided that we were ready to have a baby. After meeting with my ob-gyn, I felt defeated. He told me that because of my irregular cycles, I'd probably need fertility medications, such as Clomid, in order to conceive. Yet because of the knowledge I had gained working with WomanCode, I knew that I was ovulating. Without even taking my temperature, I knew the signs to look for—such as changes in discharge—to know what my body was doing. My husband and I decided to try to get pregnant naturally before considering medical intervention. We had sex a few times, and seven weeks later I found out I was pregnant. I truly believe that my baby was possible because of how well I came to know my own body.

Hygiene, X-Rays, Bacteria, and
Your Long-Term Fertility

When it comes to fertility, the women I work with are either actively trying to conceive or wanting to know how to preserve their fertility for when they want to become pregnant, no matter how many years that may be from now.

There is significant evidence that links chemical, radiation, and bacterial exposure to impairing fertility in the long term. There are

The Pill, STDs, and Your Fertility

*In addition to masking underlying fertility-dampening hormonal issues—issues you may not even know you have—the Pill can compromise your fertility in another way: by giving you a false sense of security with sex. I see so many women who assume that because the Pill reduces their risk of becoming pregnant, they don't need to use condoms during intercourse. At the risk of sounding like a public service announcement, the Pill does **not** protect against sexually transmitted diseases (STDs). STDs such as chlamydia and gonorrhea cause enough issues to your health on their own; but they can also contribute to pelvic inflammatory disease (PID), a "silent" condition that can permanently damage your fallopian tubes, uterus, and surrounding tissues, which in turn can result in infertility, without any warning. And while I'm all for receiving as much pleasure as possible, research shows that the more sex partners a woman has, the greater her risk of developing PID. This is because of the potential for increased exposure to infections that can cause the disease. Bottom line: unless you're in a committed, long-term, monogamous relationship and both partners have tested negative for STDs, using a condom during sex—whether or not you're on the Pill—is just one more thing you can do to safeguard your fertility.*

simple ways for you to protect your reproductive organs, hormones, and egg quality with some key lifestyle changes on top of the Woman-Code protocol. For women who want to protect their fertility, here are my top four recommendations:

- *Keep your uterus happy.* Always, always, always use a condom during intercourse. Even if you're married or in a long-term committed, monogamous relationship. *Always.* This will significantly reduce bacterial exposure in the uterus, which is a huge impediment to conception. You'll also prevent exposure to STDs, bacterial vaginosis, urinary tract infections, and chronic yeast infections, which destabilize the pH of the vagina and cause bacterial overgrowth in the uterus, which can be major hurdles—especially if these problems endure for long periods of time—when you decide that you want to become pregnant. Even if you and your partner are extremely healthy people, sperm carry microbes that can create pH imbalances in the uterus without creating any symptoms.

- *Swap toxic cleaning products for natural ones.* Do what you can to avoid exposure to endocrine disruptors. Become vigilant about the products you use in your home and on your body. These toxins can accumulate in your body and very slowly disrupt your endocrine system. Although you might not notice symptoms, they could still be wreaking havoc on your fertility that you wouldn't know about until you tried to conceive. Switch to natural cleaning products like Seventh Generation's.

- *Floss daily.* Maintain good oral hygiene. Brush twice a day, floss at least once a day, and visit your dentist every six months. A 2011 study at the University of Western Australia found that women with gum disease took an average of seven months to become pregnant—two months, on average, longer than women without gum disease. Gum disease–causing bacteria can travel in the bloodstream throughout the body and set off an inflammatory response that can harm tissues in nearly every organ, including your heart and reproductive areas. While it's important to visit your dentist regularly, decline frequent oral X-rays. Although dentists often recommend some kind of X-ray at every visit, limit them to once every two years. The small dose of radiation from the X-ray machine can, over time, harm your thyroid and alter hormone levels to a degree that can affect your fertility.

- *Safer airport security (for your ovaries).* Also decline going through the new X-ray scanning machines at airports (the regular metal detector is fine) and request a pat-down instead. The X-ray scanning machine delivers a small dose of radiation to all the organs and glands of your endocrine system and can cause damage over time. (This is especially problematic for frequent travelers.) The pat-down—which on a woman is always performed by a woman—takes only about three minutes, so schedule it into your travel time.

Conceiving should be easy, right? Instead, getting pregnant can sometimes be frustrating, scary, and stressful. In this chapter we took a holistic view of all of the factors that go into reproductive health to recognize that it's no longer something that we can just take for granted. Just like successful weight loss involves a multifaceted approach, so too does fertility. We have to be vigilant about the WomanCode protocol, reduce our exposure to endocrine disruptors, partner with our doctors to get hormonally evaluated early on, make

Bringing It Back After Baby

So much happens hormonally during pregnancy and after that it's normal to feel like your body is taking you on a ride. When eating to nourish your endocrine system, you can expect to enjoy this journey of becoming a mother. Many women, however, enter pregnancy with stressed and depleted bodies and find themselves hormonally vulnerable postpartum. They feel exhausted, depressed, and uncomfortable in their own bodies. It's interesting to trace the root of these symptoms back to food. Mood is stabilized by neurochemicals like serotonin, dopamine, and norepinephrine. Much of our serotonin is produced in our small intestine. Brain health and mental health overall are supported by key nutrients that we get from food. It's essential that you are eating for emotional wellness after baby. Consider that for nine months you have been sharing all of your micronutrients from your diet with your growing baby, and then after your child is born, you may be breast-feeding as well. Both of these physical experiences require tremendous nutritional support. All of the micronutrients needed to create your baby's healthy brain, for example, are the very same ones you need too. It's so important for women to take an excellent supplement during pregnancy but also equally important after, especially if you want to bring yourself back to a healthier hormonal state. Omega-3s, B complex, Vitamin D3, calcium, and magnesium are my top choices for women struggling with postpartum depression, exhaustion, and low sex drive as well as relying on the basics of the protocol to incorporate whole grains, good-quality fats, and fiber. These nutrients will help you improve serotonin production, nourish your overworked adrenals due to massive short-term lack of sleep, and will help promote healthy estrogen and progesterone balance. The key here is to recognize that you must feed yourself as vigilantly as you did while pregnant. You are still eating for two, just in a different way. As every mother knows, when Mama's happy and healthy, everyone is happy and healthy.

sure we are eating nutrient-dense, fertility-enhancing foods whether we are doing IVF or not, and adopt a fertile mind-set so we can turn that nurturing, maternal energy onto ourselves and so that we can see ourselves creating in other areas of our lives while our bodies become optimally primed for conception. My clients find that putting their attention on what they *can* impact greatly reduces the stress that can so often accompany fertility challenges and exacerbate the issue from an endocrine standpoint. Invest in your body, rely on the WomanCode protocol, and partner with a doctor you feel good about. You must play a role in making your body more fertile whether you choose to try conceiving naturally or use IVF.

SUCCESS STORY: Lisa Marie Rice, 36

CONDITION: Infertility, PCOS, Postpartum Depression

After I got married, it came time for us to think about starting a family. After several months of being off the Pill and not yet ovulating, I went to the ob-gyn. An ultrasound confirmed that I had PCOS. The emotional roller coaster was horrendous. I was on medication, I had injections, I was monitored daily via ultrasound, I lost my first pregnancy, and finally, after two and a half years, I was pregnant with my son. While staying home with him, I noticed the PCOS symptoms were coming back. The weight gain was stubborn and, once again, I was depressed.

I knew about FLO Living from a friend of mine and lurked on the site for several months until I decided I would sign up for a free tele-class that Alisa was giving. I really didn't know what to expect. I knew I wanted to have another child without IVF, and so I figured if I started working on this now, maybe I could cut out a lot of the pain suffered the first time around.

After completing the program, I got a period! It has been regular since then. Six months after completing the program, my skin was clear, and my blood work was normal and my ovaries were back down

One-on-One with Alisa

Let's get proactive. Are you trying to conceive now? Going through IVF? Or do you want to make sure you don't run into problems when you are ready to get pregnant? First identify the items from this chapter that need your attention. Where can you start immediately? Is it time to get rid of the laundry detergent, dryer sheets, bleach-based cleaning chemicals? Are you going to up the flossing and fertile foods? Perhaps you just need to stay focused on the protocol basics. Putting your attention there and staying out of overwhelm and stress is essential for your healthy conception.

---

to normal size. My current gynecologist was amazed! She noticed the difference as soon as she came into the examining room. While having a routine ultrasound, we learned that all of my ovarian cysts were gone. I remember the tech saying to me, "I am looking at your ovary now." I recall being confused because I could not see them. You see, I used to define my ovaries by the cysts on them. I could not find the cysts and I kept asking, "Where is my ovary?" And my husband exclaimed, "The cysts are gone!"

All of this, however, is not the amazing part of my story.

By the time my IVF-conceived son was about a year old, we started thinking of giving him a sibling. Two months after trying to conceive, we conceived our second son. We were told that we would have difficulty because of my history, but it was because I went through the FLO Living protocol that I was able to conceive so easily and quickly.

The pregnancy was extremely easy and uneventful. I didn't suffer from postpartum depression as I did with my first son, and I was able to breast-feed. Two years later, I am still eating on program and feel great.

I signed up with FLO Living expecting them to tell me how to eat so I could get healthy and have drug-free conception. I got that and more. I learned how to live a fulfilling and healthy life.

If you are actively trying to conceive, I want you to begin connecting with your uterus and ovaries. I want you to imagine that your uterus is in fact the beautiful vessel or container that it is and visualize light and energy swirling inside of this vessel. Imagine this to be the most amazing place for a new life to begin. For a few minutes before bed, close your eyes, place a hand over your lower abdomen, and do this visualization before falling asleep. This is not meant to be an esoteric exercise; you will actually be increasing blood flow to the reproductive organs by breathing deeply, and aligning your body with your intentions to conceive and become a mother.

Finally, I'd like you to pick one area of your life outside of your health, where you can express yourself creatively. What was a favorite hobby of yours as a child? Commit to doing something that feels creative for you during the next month—dancing, singing, writing, painting, crafting, cooking, playing an instrument—whatever you define as an expression of your creative energy. Observe the shifts in your energy.

CHAPTER 8

Supercharge Your Sex Drive

It's no longer only a factor of age that a woman's libido takes a nosedive. Due to all of the same stressors that are compromising your menstrual health and fertility today, your appetite for sex is also at stake. I see women as young as thirty who are struggling with sluggish energy and a barely-there libido. Like conception, most women think that sex is supposed to just happen. That with just one kiss knees should weaken; that the moment their mind wanders to sex they should feel frisky and be ready to get it on at the drop of a hat (or bra). Then, once they're having sex, they think they should be able to orgasm just as easily. And if they're not even close to climaxing in what they believe is an appropriate timeframe, they fear they're disappointing their partner. So they either fake the big O or shift their focus onto their partner's pleasure, abandoning their own entirely.

I was giving a lecture called "Hot Mama Hormones" for the Holistic Mom Network one seriously rainy night in Andover, Massachusetts. It was raining so hard, I was sure that no one would end up coming, though I had been booked two months in advance. Now for Manhattan, this combination of the timing and the weather would instantly mean a smaller crowd. To my great surprise, not only did everyone show up, but we had to bring in more chairs and by the time I got up to speak, the room was packed to standing. I had to know why! I shared with the women what I had been anticipating due to the intense weather and timing of the workshop and asked how it was that so many of these women who had jobs, kids, husbands, and homes to attend to made it out on that dark and stormy Friday night. Their collective answer truly tickled me. Their husbands had gone out of their way to cook dinner, feed the kids, and clear their calendars to support their wives in attending this seminar on recovering lost libido after baby or during motherhood. The women ranged in age from thirty to fifty and the story was the same as I asked them to share their experiences with me. They had never really recovered hormonally from pregnancy, hormonal issues that they had either not been aware of or had not had the chance to do anything about before pregnancy got worse postpartum, and now they were faced with little time and energy to do much about their missing sex drive. Although it was almost comical how the husbands were so keen to have their women get "turned back on," the women in that room wanted more. I just love how we women always want more—that energy of desire for change creates everything. These women wanted to know how to fix their bodies so they could feel more energized, have more stable moods, and enjoy their lives more fully, and yes, of course, sex and having a sex drive was a part of that. I knew I would be able to help them that night because what I had to offer in that workshop, and what I'll be offering you in this chapter, is the very same holistic view of restoring and maintaining your sex drive. It isn't just about being able to have an orgasm. It's about being able to have the energy to enjoy your life, and these women knew that a better working definition should match their intuitive desire and showed up ready to learn. I did learn later on that the husbands were very satisfied with their investment of support. I applaud their desires too—it's a smart man who knows that when his woman is happy, healthy, and fulfilled, their relationship benefits.

In my practice over the past decade, I've seen women of every age come in and want this very same thing. I'm going to map out a plan for you to keep the libido engine humming along happily throughout your life. It will of course start with expanding our understanding of our sexual response beyond what most of us glean from magazines or, even worse, pornography. I'm going to show you how to engage in different types of sex throughout your cycle so you can leverage your natural energy stores more effectively. I'll then share my favorite supplements and foods to help you kickstart your sex drive. Most importantly, I'm going to guide you to seek out daily opportunities to create pleasurable (nonsexual) experiences for yourself, to prime yourself when you so desire for the horizontal kind of pleasurable experiences.

When you look at many women's assumptions about what their sexual experience should be like, it's less expansive than it actually is. These assumptions reflect a lack of understanding about what the sexual response is and how it works—a mind-set that goes back to the static view most women have of the body: that it should perform at the same level, in the same way, every single day throughout your life. Well, I'm going to put those and many other misconceptions to rest and help you better understand the mysteries of your libido so that you can create a juicier experience in and out of the bedroom.

The most detrimental misunderstanding about your libido is that sex is all in your head. I'm so tired of women being told that their sexual response is entirely in their mind, because that's only *part* of the picture. Research has shown that a woman can view pornography of any kind—straight, gay, or animal—and her body will show all the signs of arousal. In that moment, she may not desire sex; but if she's looking at sex, her body will respond accordingly. What this means: there's a feedback loop you can work to your advantage. Yes, you can be thinking about sex and not necessarily be in the mood for sex, yet your body will be primed for it. But your body can also be primed for sex first, and when your brain receives this information it responds by creating a mental and physical state of arousal. So if you're fed up with hearing that if you'd just clear your mind of your grocery list or stop thinking about your thighs sex would be more pleasurable, you can now see that there's a whole other side to the story that you can put into action. No matter what the basis is for feeling like you're in a sexual rut today, the good news is that the body can lead the brain to an incredible sexual experience every single time. (I'll show you how in this chapter.) This is an even deeper application of what you've already been working toward—living in partnership with your body—and what could be more fun than putting it into action with sex?

Before I dive into the biology of your sexual response, I want to state up front that all the information in this chapter applies no matter what kind of relationship you're in, or if you're not in one at all. This is about *you*. The tools I'm giving you are about your enjoyment of your body. The way I see it, you can enjoy being with someone else's body only if you've been practicing how to enjoy being in your own. That's a very big distinction, because many women look at sex as a way to please their partner. But if you want to have a healthy libido, you won't be thinking about pleasing anyone but yourself. Then, when the clothes come off, *everyone* will have a richer experience because of that. The bottom line is that *you* play a huge role in how you experience your sex drive. You're responsible for turning yourself on—no one has that power but you. Others can enhance your pleasure or take it to a higher level, but the initial experience of being turned on starts with what you're doing, throughout your day, for yourself.

Your Body on Sex

Your sexual response is an amazing, highly refined process that's the result of millennia of evolutionary progress. In the 1960s two scientists, William Masters and Virginia Johnson, examined over ten thousand sexual encounters in men and women in order to delineate the exact order of events that make up the sexual response. What they found: not only is it very similar from one woman to the next, but men's and women's bodies also experience the same four stages of the sexual response:

- *Initial arousal.* Sometimes known as the excitement phase, arousal can last several minutes to several hours. Your heart rate, blood pressure, and respiration increase. Your blood vessels dilate, engorging all the tissues of your sex organs— the nipples, clitoris, labia, and vagina. Glands in your vaginal walls secrete lubricating liquid and make you feel wet.

- *Plateau.* This stage is a continuation of arousal. Your tissues swell even more. Breathing, heart rate, and blood pressure continue to rise. The clitoris becomes more sensitive. Muscles within the vagina tighten, reducing the diameter of the opening. You may moan or vocalize involuntarily.

- *Orgasm.* Vaginal lubrication increases, muscles in the vaginal walls constrict, and the overall pleasure of your body increases. If you climax in this stage—not a given (see below)—you experience quick cycles of contractions in the muscles of your pelvic floor, and you may feel muscle spasms in other areas of the body. You may have a surge of lubrication.

- **Resolution.** After climax, your muscles relax and your body releases from its aroused state.

In my view of the sexual response, the orgasmic phase and climax are two separate things. It's important to distinguish them as a way of getting to know your body even better. The orgasmic phase is the process of excitement, engorgement, and a neurochemical cascade that I'll describe in the next section of this chapter. Every woman can have an orgasmic experience even if she doesn't climax. (More on that in a moment, too.) For those women who climax, some can climax multiple times, while others experience too much clitoral sensitivity in the resolution phase to endure the amount of sensation needed to climax again. The resolution phase varies tremendously from person to person—some are immediately ready for round two, while in others the resolution period may last as long as twenty-four hours.

My point is: while all four stages occur for every woman (and man) throughout the sexual response, understanding *your* unique physiological response can be incredibly empowering. Observe what's happening in your body and work with it. Now that you know what the four stages of sexual response are, see how they feel in your own body. Do you need more time in initial arousal before penetration for the plateau and orgasmic phases to feel as mind-blowing? (Hint: most women do.) What do you feel like in the resolution phase? Are you immediately ready for sex again, or do you feel spent or übersensitive? Get to know your pleasure recipe as intimately as possible.

Just as you've come to understand your unique response to individual foods, continuously investigate your body's response to sexual stimulation. In that way you can learn what you need, from yourself or your partner, to move through all four phases of the sexual response.

If you feel like you've lost your ability to climax (or it's *always* been MIA for you), know that as you improve your hormonal balance through the WomanCode protocol, your ability to climax will improve as well. When estrogen, progesterone, and testosterone are out of balance, you lack the ideal ratios of the neurochemicals, described below, essential for a robust sexual response. Balancing your hormones and embracing your unique pleasure recipe will set the neurological and physical stage for you to have that mind-blowing climax you're after.

Your Brain on Sex

Your sexual response is no longer a mystery, but have you ever wondered what's responsible for causing the changes you experience in each stage? It'll be no surprise to learn that it all comes back to your hormones. For decades, scientists believed that sex drive was all about testosterone. However, they're now finding that estrogen and progesterone play a huge role, too. What I love about this reality is that, whereas before, when the sex response was believed to be testosterone-driven, it felt like a man's game, now it can be viewed just as much as a woman's game. In addition, we have the potential for an even more robust sexual experience because of all of our hormones. Since our hormones are cyclical and the concentrations vary throughout our menstrual cycle, sex doesn't feel the same each and every time for women as it does, more typically, for men. You're hardwired to have an abundance of experiences. How cool is that? As you learned in chapter 5, the concentrations of your different hormones determine where you are in your menstrual cycle. Since your sexual response depends on these very same hormones, their concentrations in each phase also determine your sexual response—both your mental urge and your physical ability to be aroused. (Later in this chapter I'll show you how to cross-train sex with your cycle to maximize your libido in each of the four phases of your menstrual cycle.)

In addition to the three above-named sex-related hormones (estrogen, progesterone, and testosterone), your libido is also governed by four groups of neurochemicals: neurotransmitters that target the pleasure areas of your brain (serotonin and dopamine), nitric oxide, oxytocin, and cortisol. Here are the roles each group plays when it comes to sex:

- *Pleasure chemicals.* Serotonin and dopamine target the feel-good regions of your brain. Not only do they boost your experience of pleasure; they make you want to do the behavior that elicits their release over and over again. (These are the same neurochemicals many drugs of abuse elicit, too, but to a much greater degree that can lead to addiction.) If you've ever heard that certain antidepressants dampen sex drive, that's because a certain class—those called selective serotonin reuptake inhibitors (SSRIs)—blocks serotonin's ability to bind with receptors in the brain. While this can help improve mood in people who suffer from depression, lower concentrations of serotonin in the brain can decrease sex drive (since the neurotransmitter is essential for feeling aroused).

- **Nitric oxide.** As levels of nitric oxide rise, your blood vessels relax, enabling blood to flow more efficiently through them. This vasodilation causes all the tissues in your sex organs to become engorged, heightening their sensitivity and boosting your arousal. While sexual activities certainly increase nitric oxide release, you can experience a surge of it in countless ways throughout your day. Anything that gets the blood flowing in your body, such as exercising or getting a massage, can do the trick. Of course, increased vasodilation isn't beneficial just for sex; it can improve your overall health by increasing oxygenation to your heart and brain and lowering your blood pressure.

- **Oxytocin.** You may have heard of oxytocin as the chemical that bonds new moms with their babies. A new mother's body releases huge amounts of this hormone during birth and breast-feeding. In a sexual context, it also leads to desire, can facilitate climax, and makes you feel more connected to your partner.

- **Cortisol.** You're most familiar with cortisol as the so-called stress hormone, but it impacts sex as well: all of its effects on the body when you're under stress decrease your sexual response. That's because cortisol curbs all bodily functions that are nonessential to your survival when there's a threat. Primarily, it suppresses your immune system, digestion, growth, and reproduction. It can also disrupt the menstrual cycle, which can take a toll on your sex drive. After all, from an evolutionary standpoint it would be unsafe to carry a child if your own well-being were in jeopardy.

  Cortisol also constricts blood vessels and increases blood pressure. When blood vessels narrow, they're unable to engorge and can prevent you from entering the initial arousal phase. (We women aren't the only ones who suffer—high levels of cortisol can cause erectile dysfunction and a decrease in desire for men, too.) Conversely, however, sex can be tremendously beneficial in lowering your cortisol levels. Every time you experience orgasm, your body experiences a huge cortisol flush, getting it out of your system. It may seem like a chicken-and-egg scenario (too much cortisol decreases arousal, but feeling aroused reduces cortisol), but you don't have to depend on sexual stimulation to score that cortisol drain. All the activities I focus on later in this chapter—activities designed to bring more pleasure into your life—will remove that excess cortisol so your libido can flow more freely. Bottom line: it's crucial to control cortisol levels, because a healthy amount allows you to have a robust sexual response, but too much can take a toll on your libido.

Let's recap your sexual response on a physical and neurological level. I talked about the four stages of your sexual response (arousal, plateau, orgasm, and resolution); I mentioned the three hormones involved in fueling your sex drive (testosterone, estrogen, and progesterone); and I explained the four types of neurochemicals that play a role in your libido (serotonin and dopamine, nitric oxide, oxytocin, and cortisol). Now I'm going to show you how all that fits together.

Given the fact that your hormone levels determine each of the four phases of your menstrual cycle and also play a role in your sexual response, what you do sexually in each of the four phases can elicit the optimal neurochemical cascade. While you can't control what your hormones are doing in each of the four phases of your menstrual cycle (nor should you want to), you can depend on them as a baseline and do different things sexually in order to experience a surge in serotonin, dopamine, nitric oxide, and oxytocin, as well as a flush of

SUCCESS STORY: *Fran Mooney, 48*

CONDITION: Low Libido

I originally came to the WomanCode program for the specific purpose of doing something to restore my libido and energy, which had gone missing with the onset of perimenopause. The creams and hormones weren't working for me, and I wanted to be more natural in my approach. Throughout the three-month program, I redefined my concept of sexuality, and I've fallen in love with a new way of being that has allowed me to live and love more fully every day. My husband loves it, too! I've refocused my personal goals and redefined for myself what "success" really means to me. Alisa is an amazingly wise, caring, insightful, and intuitive woman who improved my ability to change. The program more than exceeded my expectations—it made me a new woman!

cortisol. Just as you can cross-train your life with diet, exercise, and lifestyle choices to maximize your hormonal potential, you can cross-train your cycle with sex to boost your desire and physical arousal. Ladies, what I'm saying is that *you* are the creator of your libido. You can manipulate and change it in each phase of your menstrual cycle to create the most satisfying sexual experience possible.

Cycle-Sync Your Sex Drive

As promised, we'll focus now on how to optimize arousal in each of the four phases. When it comes to coping with a sex drive that has sputtered, it's often the desire piece—the *lack* of arousal—that makes you feel disconnected from your body and, as the case may be, from your partner. If you're in a place where you've healed your hormones through the WomanCode protocol, then each of the other stages of sexual response—plateau, orgasm, and resolution—will fall in line once you feel aroused. Getting to that first stage can take a special set of skills based on your hormonal ratios in each phase of your menstrual cycle. With the tools below you'll be able to ignite that initial spark.

☽ FOLLICULAR PHASE

- *Hormone focus.* Levels of estrogen, testosterone, and progesterone start at their lowest point in your cycle now, though increase toward ovulation, which means your sex drive may be at its lowest, too, depending where you are during this time.

- *Sex focus.* Pour your attention into the arousal phase in order to get to a place where you have both the mental desire and the physical urge (such as lubrication) for sex. In bed, this means lots of touching, massage, and nonpenetrating foreplay (whether you're alone or with someone else). Remember from chapter 5 how you respond to new things well in this phase? Consider massive, extended foreplay as one way of experimenting with newness, sexually, in your follicular phase.

● OVULATORY PHASE

- *Hormone focus.* Thanks to a peak in testosterone and estrogen as well as a surge in luteinizing hormone (a precursor to progesterone) and follicular-stimulating hormone, in the ovulatory phase you move into arousal without much stimulation at all. You're also most fertile in this phase, so your body is primed to crave and seek out sex at this time. And because cervical secretions throughout your ovulatory phase keep you lubricated (even though it's different from sex-related lubrication), you may move more seamlessly from arousal to plateau.

- *Sex focus.* Between your boost in desire and your naturally high energy levels in this phase, have at it! This is the time to have intense, passionate, physical sex (however you define it and enjoy it).

☾ LUTEAL PHASE

- *Hormone focus.* In the first half of the luteal phase, testosterone is still present from the ovulatory phase, while estrogen and progesterone climb to their peak. In the second half of the luteal phase, testosterone takes a dip to follicular-phase levels, and estrogen and progesterone begin to decrease.

- *Sex focus.* What this means for your sexual response is that in the first half you may still feel hot and ready for sex, but you may need more stimulation to climax in the orgasmic phase. Seek out additional stimulation as you plateau—perhaps include a vibrator or other toy to increase sensation. In the second half of this phase, you may no longer feel in the mood for sex, so spend more time in the arousal phase and look for ways to turn yourself on and increase initial excitement. With appropriate arousal, you'll soon find yourself feeling juicy and ready for more, and your physical response will reflect that.

○ **MENSTRUAL PHASE**

- *Hormone focus.* Hormone levels advance quickly to their lowest concentrations. If you have a shorter cycle and bleed heavily on the first few days, your hormones may immediately drop off and be at their lowest point. However, if you have a longer cycle with spotting at the beginning, estrogen may remain a little higher and progesterone lower at the beginning of your menstrual phase before dropping off, and you may feel more symptomatic as a result.

- *Sex focus.* Here's where the question of whether or not to have sex during your period comes into play. If you're someone who frequently experiences yeast infections or urinary tract infections, you may want to steer clear of sex during menstruation, because low pH levels in your vagina at this time can increase your susceptibility to bacteria. For women with symptomatic cycles, your unbalanced hormone levels may make you feel uninterested in sex during your period—and that's okay. Just as it's a good idea to take time away from other physical activities and give your body a rest during this phase, it can also be a time when you abstain from sex for a few days. Still, there are plenty of women who find that sex relieves their menstrual cramps and migraines and who enjoy the different sensations they feel when having sex during their period. Let your body be your guide.

Using Sex to Heal Your Hormones

If you're reading this book because you have menstrual or fertility issues, then cross-training your sexual experiences with your cycle

Top-Ten Health Benefits of Sex for Women

- *Improves circulation to organs in the pelvic cavity, delivering nutrients, growing healthy tissues, and regulating the menstrual cycle. Women who have intercourse at least once a week are more likely to have normal menstrual cycles than women who are celibate or who have infrequent sex.*

- *Increases fertility and a sense of wellness by energizing the hypothalamus gland (which regulates appetite, body temperature, and emotions) and the pituitary gland (which in turn regulates the release of reproductive hormones that induce ovulation and cervical fluid).*

- *Provides overall lymphatic massage, helping the body's natural detoxification process to improve digestion and mood and help prevent cancer.*

- *Promotes healthy estrogen levels to keep vaginal tissues supple and protect against osteoporosis and heart disease.*

- *Induces deep relaxation by boosting endorphin levels and flushing cortisol out of the body.*

- *Spikes levels of nitric oxide, a "miracle molecule," and DHEA, a hormone that improves brain function, balances the immune system, helps maintain and repair tissue, and promotes healthy skin.*

- *Helps a woman look younger. Studies show that making love three times a week in a stress-free relationship can make you look ten years younger.*

- *Boosts infection-fighting cells up to 20 percent—helps fight colds and flu!*

- *Cures migraines and helps treat other types of pain by elevating pain thresholds (a bonus when preparing for childbirth!).*

- *Increases levels of the hormone oxytocin, which is linked to passion, intuition, and social skills—the hormone of bonding and success!*

can be an enormously beneficial piece of the hormone-healing puzzle. For starters, sex (alone or with a partner) provides all the advantages listed in the "Top-Ten Health Benefits of Sex" sidebar— advantages that improve the overall state of your endocrine system. In addition, syncing your cycle with sex keeps your adrenal glands

Sex in Your Postmenopausal Years

If you're in your postmenopausal years, while you are not still cycling, you can lean into the blueprint to bring a fresh approach to your activities. And I'm going to let you in on a little secret that does not get nearly the airtime it should: a woman's sex drive is meant to increase over time and it's actually **easier** to work with your libido after menopause. This may seem counterintuitive, but it's because you don't have as many hormonal fluctuations to consider. You have one consistent estrogen-testosterone-progesterone cocktail that's lower than in menstruating women but that very much reflects the lower levels of that cocktail in the follicular phase of the menstrual cycle. Therefore, just as in the follicular phase, your attention, energy, and focus should go toward the arousal stage of your sexual response.

Set the expectation for yourself that the purpose is not to "finish" but to maximize pleasurable sensations of any and all kinds. Take all the time that you need to enjoy yourself. This can include how you delight all of your senses throughout the day well before a sexual encounter. Expand your definition of pleasure.

Now that you know the role these hormones play in creating your sexual response, you can see why it's so important to spend as much time as possible not only in foreplay, but also in seeking out pleasurable experiences throughout your day. (Read more about this in the section headed "Turning Yourself On," below.) With some sensual experimentation (the best kind of research!), you can find out what it takes for you to reach the arousal stage and create an even richer sex life.

healthy. In addition to the huge cortisol flush that sweeps the stress hormone out of your body during arousal and sex, the different recommendations I made (above) for each phase sync up with the energy you feel mentally and physically. This means that you can use sex to *support* your adrenals instead of *draining* them. That's why I suggest experimenting with intense, energetic sex in the ovulatory phase when your energy is higher, rather than during your menstrual phase when rest may be what your body needs most.

Turning Yourself On

Many people think about their libido solely in terms of what's happening (or not happening, as the case may be) in their bedroom. But I like to use a broader definition of the word: your ability to give and receive pleasure, enjoyment, and acknowledgment. With this definition in mind, try thinking about your libido in a new way: in order for you to feel turned on in bed, you need to feel turned on during your daily life. Part of the problem is that when you hear the word *pleasure,* you probably think about sensual pleasure. What I'd like you to think about instead is pleasing your senses all day. It's enormously difficult to fully surrender to pleasure during sex—or even to *want* sex—if the pleasure in your life has run dry. If you're tired, overextended, or burned out, I'm sure you know exactly what I'm talking about. Your energy and your libido are directly related. Working forty-plus hours a week while juggling a social life or even kids and a family makes it nearly impossible to feel the pulse of libido in your everyday life. But I'm going to show you how to reclaim that pleasure.

Let's begin with your frame of mind. I know that you're busy and that your responsibilities often make you feel like you're supposed to accomplish thirty hours' worth of activities within a twenty-four-hour timeframe. But imagine for a moment that you didn't have to change anything about what you needed to do, and altered only your approach to *what you're already doing*. Namely: going about your day with more pleasure. It's what I call the vitality mind-set. At its crux is this question: How can you find more enjoyment in everyday things?

Say, for instance, that you needed to send dozens of work-related e-mails after you got home from work at night. You could choose to put your nose to the grindstone and power through the list feeling frustrated, overwhelmed, and resentful. Or you could light a few

Create Your Pleasure Recipe

You can extend the initial arousal phase for hours before sex is even a question (and afterward, too). Working the activities listed below into your daily, weekly, or monthly schedule will infuse your days with pleasure and create a neurochemical balance in your brain that makes it easier to relish your experience in that first stage of excitement.

- *Remove things and activities that drain your adrenals. Take a break from stimulants, such as coffee, for at least a month and see how you feel. Aim for thirty to forty-five minutes of physical activity such as walking per day, but avoid intense exercise such as kickboxing, or sprinting, which the body interprets as a stressor.*

- *Take two supplements daily: vitamin C with bioflavonoids and ashwagandha. Both of these help heal the adrenal tissues and boost adrenal function.*

- *Schedule five to ten minutes of relaxing activity before bed each day. Examples: apply skin care products, read, meditate.*

- *Schedule thirty minutes of self-pleasure once a week. Try using only your hands and fingers for a better tumescent experience than using toys, in order to get the most nitric oxide benefits for your body.*

candles, put on some music, change into something comfortable, and try to enjoy the process as much as possible. You could also seek out chances to connect with the people you're writing to by choosing words that communicate your passion about what you're doing. These are tiny shifts that can cause a significant transformation in how you live your life and how you experience libido in mundane activities.

Enhancing the quality of each day isn't about leading to sex as much as it is about cultivating pleasure so that your daily life isn't as draining on a physical, emotional, and hormonal scale. And now that you know about the biology of your sex drive, it's incredible to see the difference these small things make in moving you into the initial

- *Schedule thirty minutes to do nothing once a week. Minimize stimulation. Take a nap. Sit outside surrounded by trees and nature.*

- *Add plenty of healthy fats to your diet. Try avocados, oils, nuts, and seeds to support the organs of your reproductive system.*

- *Fill your diet with foods that nurture the adrenals. To recharge your energy, go heavy on blue/black and yellow/orange foods (see below), which represent water and earth in Chinese medicine—two important qualities for enhancing energy and libido.*

Blue/Black Foods	Yellow/Orange Foods
Black beans	Carrots
Black sesame seeds	Oranges
Adzuki beans	Sweet potatoes
Sea vegetables (such as seaweed) and water chestnuts	Apricots
Dark chocolate	Squash and pumpkin

arousal state. Every time you experience pleasure in your day, your sex-related neurochemicals are affected in some way—serotonin, dopamine, and nitric oxide are released; whenever you feel close to someone, you experience an oxytocin surge. *All* of these activities result in a cortisol flush. In other words, the more pleasure you infuse into your day, the more your body is primed for arousal.

If you want to better understand what libido outside the bedroom looks like, look no further than food. There's a reason why people are drawn to watching the Food Network round-the-clock (hello, food porn!). Each chef completely embodies turn-on—they're pursuing something they're passionate about, enjoying every miniscule detail of what they're doing (as simple as it may be), and thriving on the opportunity to share their passion with others. Or if you ever visit a farmers' market, pause in your shopping and look around. You'll see people engaging their arousal phase at every turn—smelling foods, feeling them, tasting them, and talking about them. Since food is such a multisensory experience, it's one of the easiest ways to begin experimenting with your everyday libido. (Taking the time to eat mindfully and slowly can also help prevent overeating, improve digestion, and help your body absorb nutrients—a wonderful added bonus.) If you're someone who enjoys cooking or you're just learning to cook, begin finding the pleasure not only in the end result, but throughout the entire process—from making your grocery list, to shopping, to cooking, to serving the food and eating it. It's an experience that lends itself to so many opportunities for pleasure that you'll be amazed at how energized you feel by the time you put a meal on the table. And that's exactly what a healthy libido is all about! If you feel exhausted and drained at the end of the day, you've likely gone through it with no turn-on. But if you seek out those little moments of pleasure, you're going to find yourself feeling more relaxed and at ease when you finally get a chance to unwind.

To Give and Receive

Let's circle back to that new definition of libido: your ability to give and receive pleasure. You already saw what a difference it can make when you take an active role in giving yourself pleasure, but there's another component—receiving pleasure—that's crucial to a healthy libido. From a completely biological standpoint, the man derives his pleasure from giving and the woman experiences pleasure from receiving. But what I've noticed, in general, is that most women don't feel comfortable receiving. I've met women who won't have company over to their home unless they're able to provide refreshments, look fabulous, and decorate the living room. They'd rather not receive the pleasure of their company at all if they feel they have nothing to give. For most women, our difficulties with receiving stem from the messages we've inherited from the women in our lives who've shaped our beliefs about rest, self-indulgence, pleasure, and play.

So take a moment to think about how *you* give and receive in your life and how the ratios of each component play out. Expand your inquiry further and try this "receiving investigation"—one that I use in one-on-one sessions at FLO Living: identify five close friends and family members and ask them how they observe you *giving* support and pleasure in your relationship with them, and how they observe you *receiving* support and pleasure from them. An astounding 99 percent of the time, the data women bring back to me when they've completed this task suggest that they're not so great at the second part of this equation. It's logical that if you're not able to receive in social relationships when your clothes are on, you might find it immensely challenging to let go and receive (or even crave the act of receiving) in a sexual context with your partner when your clothes are off.

One way to begin enhancing your ability to receive is to take advantage of the generous offers people make each day. When you really pay attention, you may soon realize that those opportunities to receive crop up more frequently than you imagined. *Notice* when they're happening, and instead of reacting with a knee-jerk "No thanks" or agreeing to let someone help while plotting what you'll do to give back before you've even received, just say yes. Allow your partner to rub your shoulders. Say okay when your girlfriend offers to pick up the tab at lunch. Let another mom take over carpooling duties for the day. It's so simple, yet so powerful, to learn what receiving feels like and the many ways in which it can bring you pleasure— especially in the form of time and energy.

When women get into bed with their partner, they often don't get what they need because they're bringing the perspective that they're responsible for the other person's pleasure. But shifting your focus from giving pleasure to receiving it can be hugely transformational. It's crucial to realize that as you advance through your adult life, receiving becomes even more important to a fulfilling sexual experience; you may need to receive in more ways and take more time to receive than you used to. And that's okay. As a teenager or even in your early twenties, you probably found sex an explosive experience. You most likely didn't need much stimulation to climax. But that changes throughout your lifetime. Thus your needs, when it comes to sex, change as well. Sex becomes not just a physical sensation–seeking experience, but a means of connecting, too.

If you're hormonally compromised, you may notice that you're not achieving your maximum level of pleasure anymore, or only rarely. Rest assured, it's not only that you're tired; likewise, it doesn't mean that there's something wrong with you or with your relationship. It's simply the biological fact that the process of tumescence and engorgement takes longer and requires more mental and physical stimulation if the overall endocrine system is taxed. Maybe you need a bath, candles, and clean sheets before being able to receive sexual pleasure at this point in your life, especially if you have children—so go ahead and take a bath, light some candles, and change your sheets. It's not about becoming high-maintenance; you want more because you want to *feel* more, and all of these things will help you enter the initial arousal phase more easily and release the neurochemicals essential for arousal, engorgement, and a fulfilling sexual encounter. So do whatever is necessary to create an environment that welcomes that level of pleasure into your life. Create a setting where you can let go of everything around you and receive the pleasure that your partner is offering in that moment. And don't forget about continuing to be committed to that growing partnership with your cycling body (through each of the four phases) by engaging the sex-based tools I described earlier.

· ·

The Ten WomanCode Keys to Healthy Sexual Self-Expression

- *Living in sync with your hormones*

- *Maintaining health of your reproductive and sexual organs*

- *Managing stress to balance adrenal health and improve libido*

- *Discovering your healthy balance of masculine/feminine energetics*

- *Opening to receiving pleasure and nurturing from others*

- *Giving pleasure and nurturing to others, in a balanced way*

- *Developing healing beliefs about being a woman*

- *Moving beyond limiting beliefs about your desired sexual partner*

- *Actively pursuing your preferences and creating desires*

- *Developing and nurturing your sense of play and adventure in life*

··

The Pill and Your Libido

*One common side effect of the birth control pill is that it can dampen your libido. A 2006 study published in the **Journal of Sexual Medicine** found that birth control pills significantly decrease circulating levels of testosterone. In my experience, women who are hormonally sensitive are more likely to experience this effect, because they already have other libido-draining factors at play. During a normal menstrual cycle you typically experience two surges of testosterone that juice up your desire for sex—one during ovulation, and the other within the luteal phase. However, with the Pill, you may not experience these libido-boosting spikes. My WomanCode Rx: if you're experiencing difficulty with your libido and are currently on the Pill, consider going off it as one way to recover your thirst for pleasure.*

One-on-One with Alisa

Whether you're working to restore a low libido or want to create the richest sexual experience possible, developing a regular self-pleasure practice is extremely important. You'll build trust and confidence that your body will respond to stimulation. You'll train your brain to release the correct neurochemicals in response to your stimulation. You'll discover your personal pleasure recipe that you can call into action any time you want. You'll reap all of the physical and mental benefits that come with regular sex, such as a surge of oxytocin and nitric oxide plus a flush of cortisol. Here's how to do it.

If you're starting at zero—you rarely or never self-pleasure—start by building thirty minutes into your week, every week, for that pastime. Gradually work up to two thirty-minute sessions per week, and then increase the length of each session to as long as you can—ideally, an hour or more. Start by doing whatever you need to do to feel calm, centered, and turned on: light some candles, turn on the music, and get horizontal, whether that's in bed or in a warm bath.

Spend the first fifteen minutes staying away from your nipples, areolae, and clitoris. Stimulate other erogenous areas, such as the inner thighs, abdomen, hips, inner forearms, and upper chest, with your hands. Borrow tantric techniques: fire touch (a soft, plucking-like upward motion) and water touch (a smooth, undulating rub).

Then approach the clitoris. Using an aloe-based lubricant like Aloecadabra (nontoxic and hypoallergenic), spend as much time as you can experiencing the plateau phase and creating a building orgasmic sensation instead of focusing on climax. Touch all the different areas of your clitoris. Some women experience a lot of sensation in the upper-left quadrant, while the upper-right quadrant is more sensual for others. What feels best to you? Try different types of touch: work from bottom to top, make small circles or bigger circles, touch slowly, and touch quickly. Explore the inner labia and all the areas around your clitoris.

When you feel like you're ready to climax, use your hands or a vibrator for those final few minutes. If you opt for a vibrator, use it on the lowest setting. You'll see that you need much less stimulation when you've worked yourself into this highly aroused state. Finally, after climax, allow yourself a proper resolution phase. Relax as if you were in Savasana (the so-called corpse pose) at the end of a yoga class. Close your eyes and put one hand on your heart and one hand on your lower belly. Breathe and be with yourself for a few minutes to soak in all the sensations you created.

CHAPTER 9

Commit to the Feminine Force Within

When I was working on my own health and putting my healing protocol together, I was surprised to find that there was so much of an emotional component to achieving a state of FLO. Creating a new relationship with my body and my hormones also meant that I had some emotional cleanup to do. I had to learn to replace my inner critical voice with an inner cheerleader, to evaluate and shift the way I was engaging in relationships, and to practice trusting, receiving, and being present. Dr. Northrup, in her groundbreaking book, *Women's Bodies, Women's Wisdom*, explained that the physical symptoms I was experiencing as a woman came from the unconscious beliefs I had about being a woman. This is true not only for women suffering from PCOS, but also for those dealing with absolutely any hormonal condition.

I had never before inquired what kinds of unconscious thoughts and beliefs I had about being a woman. At that moment, for the first time,

I started to think about the messages I'd received from my own family growing up. I had incredibly supportive parents, but I remembered overhearing various family members sharing their work stories with me as I was growing up, about women at work who would talk about their hormones or PMS as a way to excuse other work issues they were having. My father felt this was not likely the best approach. He wanted me to be the best I could possibly be, no matter what. He was concerned that the world treated women differently, and he wanted me to be able to navigate a path successfully throughout my lifetime and in whatever career I chose. With my limited childhood perspective, I made an unconscious decision to adopt behaviors that were masculine, as I observed them, and to disassociate myself from being female in order to succeed. I was, and am, hardly alone in that. Every woman I've worked with can identify herself somewhere along that spectrum of trying to be "one of the guys" at some point in her life, whether it's on the sports field, in the classroom, or in the boardroom.

I came to embrace Dr. Northrup's message that the collective unconscious beliefs we carry within us about being women can, over time, influence our bodies. And if you've ever experienced a state of hormonal breakdown like the one I had, these beliefs may have taken even deeper root within you because of a sense of betrayal by your female body. When I finally connected these dots, I asked myself, *Do I really want to continue thinking this way? Do I want to see my body as a liability?* I came to see that in order for me to stick with the first four steps of the protocol and truly live in partnership with my body for the rest of my life, I had to make peace with the fact that my body is female on a very fundamental level. It wasn't enough for me to try to convince myself of this. I had to see what it was about the feminine dimension that I could *embrace, embody,* and *celebrate.*

I launched into what became two years' worth of investigating the distinction between masculine and feminine energetics. I researched all that gender psychology had to teach me on the subject and learned about Tantra—an Eastern philosophy that believes the universe is created by and made up of masculine (Shiva) and feminine (Shakti) energies that infuse all things. I then took this information and put together an understanding of masculine and feminine energy that was more practical for me and that I could share with others. The first thing I realized was that being a man or a woman doesn't give a person more or less access to masculine or feminine energy. Both energies exist within each of us in varying amounts. Learning how to engage both fully is what ends up making a person psychologically, emotionally, and physically well. Just as you wouldn't operate a remote control with only one battery, you need both of these energies as your power sources. They're necessary tools for shaping your life. Here's what masculine and feminine energy look like in action.

Masculine Energy

- Tenaciously pursuing what you want

- Deciding when/where/how a project grows

- Focusing on the end result, less on process

- Focusing on one thing at a time

- Relying on only yourself and your individual achievements

- Setting boundaries around emotions and body in order to accomplish goals

- Relating through camaraderie, entertainment, and problem solving

Feminine Energy

- Magnetically attracting what you want

- Holding the space for projects to develop at their natural pace

- Enjoying the process of creation independent of the end result

- Seeing the big picture; multitasking on many aspects of life

- Working with others; effortlessly creating community

- Connecting to emotional and physical life as a catalyst for change and development

- Relating to others by listening, sharing, and nurturing

Many of us get out of balance by focusing on or valuing one type of energy over the other. In most instances, I've found that women—especially those who've experienced hormonal breakdown—overly rely on our masculine energy and underutilize our feminine energy. Here's what I notice in women who've lost touch with their feminine energy.

Signs of Excess Masculine Energy in Women

- Feeling significant disconnection from your emotions and sensations

- Locating a sense of self-worth outside of yourself—based on material success in the world and the opinions of others

- Finding it difficult to give and receive nurturing and intimacy, including pleasure during sex

- Having fewer verbal skills for building deep relationships with friends, family, and romantic partners

- Being unable to fully get projects up and running the way you envision them

- Feeling isolated and unsupported

Once I observed that I had an energetic imbalance in my life, I examined every aspect of my day to see which energy source I was operating from at that moment. It came as no surprise that I was in my masculine mode *all day long:* at work, in my friendships, in my relationships with my family, in my self-care routine, and in the romantic relationship I was in at the time. When I saw the value of engaging my feminine energy and creating opportunities in my life to do so, I began working on the balance I exerted in all areas of my life. I actually ended the romantic relationship because my partner was unwilling to work with me to improve our dynamic—that is, our respective exchange of masculine and feminine energy. Yes, I ended a relationship because of masculine/feminine imbalance— that's how important it is! Our dynamic was never going to shift and so I had to get out for my own health and well-being, because the existing dynamic was taking a toll on my ability to thrive in every area of my life.

In fact, my team and I operate our business leveraging the intrinsic multitasking afforded us by following a pattern of cyclicality and the harmony created with embodied feminine energy. We do this on two levels. On the company-wide level, we all agree on a monthly work plan that has us starting out in the first week of the month with initiating new projects (follicular phase inspired). The second week of the month we make sure to build ample collaboration, brainstorming time (ovulatory phase inspired) in to give each project the best chance possible to get completed by the end of the month. During the third week of the month, we check in on relevant reporting, systems, customer service, and operations (luteal phase inspired) to make sure everything is going well or to bring our focused energy to things that need our attention. And in the fourth week, we have a monthly wrap-up and monthly plan-ahead meeting (menstrual phase inspired) to evaluate our progress against our planning and to affirm the best next steps.

The second way we engage this practice is on an individual level. We each engage the WomanCode protocol and are committed to living in our respective FLO, so we manage our individual menstrual cycles and energy shifts as we construct and manage our individual project execution against the company's collective plan. This practice may sound dramatic or contrived; however, in my experience of running a business for a decade, it not only helps me and the FLO Living team to stay on top of things that need our attention, to execute, and to engage our creativity without too much overwhelm. It also supports our collective desire to leverage our bodies for success. This is not to say that we don't use our masculine energy, because we most definitely do—everyone and every company must find its own best balance. I would say, for example, that Zappo's provides a most notable example of feminine-based business in action. With their extremely intimate and nurturing customer service and their collaborative and pleasure-oriented corporate culture, they are very directed in engaging as much feminine energy as possible, and what wonderful success they have created as a result.

We don't want to work from the neck up, as we believe that would be like trying to turn a TV on with a remote that has only one battery. If you had two great sources of power—your mind and your body—it seems more ridiculous to try to leave your body behind as you go through your day at work. An exclusively masculine approach would be exclusively focused on outcomes and not on the experience of customers. Employees would be multitasking at high levels, which, especially for a small business, doesn't leave much room for creativity and collaboration. Embracing this feminine energy model while growing FLO Living has shown me just how powerful and expansive feminine energy can be.

What Is Your Masculine/Feminine Balance?

Now it's your turn to identify your personal energetic balance. Think of how you typically proceed through your day. As you approach the scenarios presented, ask yourself, *Am I using masculine or feminine energy in this situation?* Then use the checklist below to reflect back on your behavior. For each item listed, check off which approach is more like you most of the time. When you've responded to all the statements, record your total number of checkmarks next to "masculine" and checkmarks next to "feminine." Are you out of balance?

Morning Routine

❑ *Masculine. You mentally review your goals for the day and plan out how you're going to accomplish them all. You try to stick to your schedule like clockwork, yelling at the kids to keep them on time, tossing sandwiches into bags, and running out the door. By the time you're dropping the kids off at school and/or sitting down at your desk, you're not even sure how you got there. The morning is a blur.*

❑ *Feminine. You wake up and take stock of how you're feeling today. You take time to do something to nurture yourself—taking a few deep breaths, doing a short meditation, or enjoying a warm shower. You make sure you connect emotionally to the people in your household—hugging the kids, kissing your partner, or chatting with your roommate. As you go about your morning routine, you check in with yourself about how you're feeling and get an intuitive sense of what you need to do to work at your best today.*

In the Thick of Your Day

❑ *Masculine. You focus on your to-do list and take the next steps right away to keep up your momentum. You push yourself and others to finish every task.*

❑ *Feminine. You reflect on the big picture, intuit what task is needed next, and trust that everything will come together. You prioritize based on what tasks will have the most value and impact for you today.*

Social Engagements

❑ *Masculine. When you're with others, you don't share what's going on; you internalize your problems until you figure out a solution. You don't want or need others' opinions because you rely on your own judgment about what's best for you.*

❑ *Feminine. You feel comfortable sharing freely about how you're feeling, and you're open to hearing supportive input from others.*

Meals

❏ *Masculine.* You eat what's in front of you, forget to eat because you're too focused on other tasks, or rigidly adhere to a diet plan even if it makes you feel hungry and depleted.

❏ *Feminine.* You plan your day ahead of time, making sure you have the food you need at hand when you'll need it. You anticipate what your body needs to prevent blood sugar crashes given your schedule for the day. You observe the signs your body gives you about your hunger levels and blood sugar and respond with appropriate food choices.

Exercise

❏ *Masculine.* You select your workout based on your fitness goals for the month. You push through no matter what.

❏ *Feminine.* You choose your workout based on how you're feeling right now. You do it to the best of your ability and do only what your body is capable of at the moment.

Time with Your Romantic Partner

❏ *Masculine.* You want to talk about what you accomplished today and then crash in front of the TV.

❏ *Feminine.* You want to talk about how you're feeling and how the people in your household are doing. You make time to connect, whether cooking and sitting down to dinner together, going for a shared walk, or spending time nestled close to your partner in bed before going to sleep.

Winding Down for the Day

❑ *Masculine.* *You organize the house, do the last bit of laundry, make your next day's to-do list, and take care of anything else you can to make sure you have a focused start tomorrow.*

❑ *Feminine.* *You look for opportunities to connect with your children, your partner, and yourself. You choose soothing activities toward the end of the day, such as reading or taking a bath.*

TOTALS: Masculine _____   Feminine _____

If you scored high in the masculine energy category, don't worry; most women I work with do. In this chapter I put a heavy focus on upping your feminine energy because so many of us rely disproportionately on our masculine side. Please keep in mind that the goal is not to live in your feminine dimension alone; rather, it's to achieve a balance and consciously use both masculine and feminine in every situation, as appropriate. Often, the best way to arrive at your own perfect balance is to start by turning up the volume on the dimension that is currently underutilized, which is what I'm encouraging you to do. This will also enable you to clearly identify the differences that tapping into your feminine energy creates in your life, since you're altering only one part of the equation.

Now that you've taken the opportunity to observe your energy ratio throughout your day, try experimenting with the different scenarios above and playing with the feminine energy experience. What might upping your feminine energy look like? Instead of multitasking at night to prepare for the next day (masculine), take time to read a book with your kids or on your own (feminine). Try it for one evening and see how you feel. At first your mind may tell you that if you don't make the next day's sandwiches at night or hammer out that to-do list, the next morning will be a disaster; you will have "wasted" time relaxing and connecting instead of preparing. What you'll find, however, is that when you spend time in your feminine dimension, you create space— space to be with your kids, space to be with your partner, space to be with yourself, space to have better-quality sleep, and space to allow your adrenals to recover. You create space to get out of your head and into your heart, and space to experience more pleasure.

After an evening powered by feminine energy, you'll wake up the next day feeling more refreshed, focused, and centered. Instead of your normal morning routine, which makes you feel like you're racing against the clock, you'll feel as if you have more time to pack those lunches, get everyone ready, and leave the house in a calm and grounded state. In other words, engaging your feminine energy creates time in the form of energy. Try this in other areas of your life as well, and ask yourself, *What improves when I'm in my feminine energy?* The answer to this question may propel you to seek ways to increase your feminine energy quotient in *every* aspect of your life.

The WomanCode Protocol: Step 5—Healing Through Feminine Energy

I never imagined partnering up with feminine energy to the fifth step—or any part—of my protocol. For a long time I thought that discovering and applying the *physical* approach to healing my body was enough. But I've found through the years that when women are feeling healthy, which the first four steps of the protocol accomplish, they gain access to a major transformative power in their life. They begin to see that, because working with their uniquely female hormones is what enabled them to heal hormonally in the first place, there must be something extraordinary about those aspects that make someone a woman. This is where my mental shift about being a woman began to take hold. I realized that embracing my feminine energy was essential to keeping myself healthy forever.

For many women, an overreliance on masculine energy is what leads to hormonal breakdown in the first place. Masculine energy and its drive to get things done despite your body can lead you to skip meals, binge on sweets, push yourself too hard at the gym, stay too long at work, and sacrifice sleep. This, as we have seen in earlier chapters, can destabilize your blood sugar, fry your adrenals, and expose you to things that clog your pathways of elimination. Masculine energy can cause you to ignore your menstrual cycle as much as possible or silence it with hormonal contraceptives in an attempt to push your body to be the same every single day. When you're relying on masculine energy, you experience a disconnection from and a disassociation with your female body.

This is why turning up the volume on your feminine energy is so crucial to your healing. It allows you to switch from *retroactively* fixing the effects of poor food, exercise, and lifestyle choices after you experience hormonal breakdown, to *proactively* making endocrine-supportive decisions to prevent hormonal breakdown. To embrace feminine energy is to live in partnership with your body. Feminine energy puts you in a mind-set of acknowledging that your body works in a cyclical fashion and encourages you to trust that it has the answers you need to continue feeling well. Even more exciting is that taking on this step of the WomanCode protocol ensures that you will have much less chance of self-sabotaging your health and self-care because you will become focused on using this energy as a tool to transform other areas of your life!

The Principles of Feminine Energy

Earlier I mentioned that it wasn't enough for me to convince myself that being a woman was a privilege and a blessing. I had to discover what it was about my feminine side that was worth committing myself to for the future. So I created tools to reprogram that deep unconscious part of my mind so I could see just how feminine energy is an extremely powerful and valuable source. This became FLO Living's Seven Principles of Feminine Energy listed below. I encourage you to engage them in situations throughout your day. Below, I offer exercises for each principle—exercises that will strengthen your relationship with your feminine energy so you can experience the opportunities which that energy creates in your life.

1. The Principle of Living in Harmony with My Biochemistry and Self-Care

I am a woman. I work with my cycle, trust the flow of change, and use each cyclical phase to create health and success. I hear my inner wisdom and practice a high level of guilt-free self-care every day.

- *Engage the principle.* Follow the first four steps of the protocol every single day.

2. The Principle of 360-Degree Emotional Expression

I celebrate my moods and emotions, including fear, anger, and sadness. I feel each feeling, learn its message, express it, and release it.

- *Engage the principle.* When someone asks you how you're doing, eliminate the response "Fine" from your vocabulary. Give a real answer that accurately describes how you're feeling in that moment.

3. The Principle of Pleasure

Sensual pleasure is a key ingredient in my daily health plan. I create situations that delight my senses and welcome moments of serendipitous pleasure, spontaneity, and fun each day.

- *Engage the principle.* Create opportunities to experience all of your senses throughout the day, in order to expand your initial arousal phase outside the bedroom. Pause and notice something outside that's visually beautiful to you. Listen to music you enjoy. Take in the aroma of your food before you eat. Hug at least one person each day. The more you intentionally work toward engaging your senses, the more you'll naturally seek opportunities to do so each day. Why? Because it feels so good!

4. The Principle of Leadership

I speak up, follow my heart, and adore my uniqueness.

- *Engage the principle.* Every day for thirty days write down at least one thing that made you feel excited, passionate, turned on, or invested in life. At the end of the month read through your list and identify whether there's a trend uniting your passions. Then look for some way—no matter how big or small—to honor the passion. It could be through volunteering, beginning a project, connecting with new people, starting a blog, creating a business, or whatever else might strike your fancy.

5. The Principle of Conscious, Collaborative Relationships

My relationships exist to support me. When old ways of relating stop working, I create new dynamics and connections. I nurture other people when doing so energizes me, not out of guilt or to obtain love or approval. I set appropriate boundaries so I can enjoy giving nurture without exhausting myself.

- ***Engage the principle.*** When leaving social encounters, check in with yourself and notice how you feel. Are you energized? Supported? Or do you feel hurt and depleted? If it's the latter, you need to set boundaries with the other person. The next time you speak to him or her, say, "It bothers me when you do X. Please don't do it again." Seek out opportunities to spend time with those who keep you feeling supported and happy. Collaboration should feel natural and effortless when you're together.

6. The Principle of Receiving

I am designed to receive. I expect, attract, seduce, welcome, and make room for love and success in my life. I believe in being supported and inviting abundance.

- ***Engage the principle.*** Give someone the opportunity to support you each day. Ask your kids to set the dinner table. Ask your partner to fold the laundry. Allow someone at work to assist you in a task. And enjoy it!

7. The Principle of Being My Own Authority

I make choices based on my body, my needs, my desires, and my inner wisdom. I believe that my body and intuition show me my true purpose, my deepest desires, and my path to wellness. I value this wisdom and access it daily.

- ***Engage the principle.*** For one week take an information vacation. Avoid those things that typically leave you feeling "less than," such as social media, tabloids, or reality TV, so that you can hear yourself and your own opinions more clearly. When you reencounter these sources after your break, you'll have a better vantage point and be able to avoid the "hypersuck" FLO Blocker that they can create. Try meditating and journaling for five minutes each day.

Rebirthing Yourself Continuously

It isn't enough for me just to help you get well. When you put down this book, I want you to feel the hugeness of your appetite for life and begin to engage in your world more fully than ever before. This requires tapping into the incredibly powerful source of feminine energy that's within you. When I started engaging my feminine energy in a deep and meaningful way, I was amazed by the number of changes that created in my body, in my work, in my relationships, and in every other aspect of my life. I see this in my clients all the time, too, as they begin to embrace their feminine energy. It became obvious to me that it's our nature, as women, to continuously create.

Your WomanCode is the mechanism for transformation in your life. Your ability to grow, evolve, and move forward in your life is due to the fact that your endocrine system, when correctly managed, functions in this way. If you've suffered a state of hormonal collapse, then you may have also experienced feelings of stagnation or a lack of momentum. Yet from your head to your ovaries a healthy endocrine system sets you up to have a dynamic, ever-changing hormonal pattern that we call the menstrual cycle. That cyclical brain and body chemistry gives you a different energy and way of being in the world from one week to the next. Even if you don't want to think your period affects your life, it does—and it does this in the best possible way. Your hormones and your menstrual cycle make you behave in a constantly dynamic way. When you engage your WomanCode and live in the FLO, you have the ability to harness that energy in order to transform your life in any way that you choose.

You were born with a physical container inside your body—your uterus—that gives birth to new life. Your hormones move through a beautiful, dynamic cycle every single month. Your whole being—your physical body, your endocrine system, and your energetic state—has hardwired you to engage in the creation process over and over again throughout your lifetime. So whether or not your health is functioning as you'd like it to, whether or not you have menstrual, fertility, or libido issues, whether or not you have a uterus, and whether or not you've ever given birth doesn't matter. As a female, you were born with this beautiful potential for creation and change.

What does this state of continuous creation look like? Often it starts with a feeling—a feeling that something's not working for you or a feeling of desire. Sometimes you may feel an urge for something more, something new, something bigger, something different. Whether you're conscious of it or not, you start asking yourself, *What do I desire? What needs to happen to satisfy this yearning?* Perhaps it's starting a new relationship, moving to a different city, going back to school, changing your career, or starting a new business. These are some of the most noticeable changes you could make, but your transformative act doesn't need to be as significant as these. It could be as simple as getting a new haircut, seeking a promotion, updating your wardrobe, redecorating your living room, starting a supper club with your friends, or adopting a pet. Once you get clear on the vision you have for change in your life, you begin to take directed, focused, and powerful action to bring that desire to life. It often starts small and gets bigger over time. This process isn't something you have to *struggle* to do. It's something you feel *compelled* to do.

I can still recall the first time I was able to identify my innate need to create change. I had experienced the feeling countless times before, but until that point I lacked a framework in which to understand it. I told a friend that I felt as if I were wearing a sweater that was too tight. What I was doing at the time career-wise didn't feel like it fit anymore. This conversation kicked off a four-year journey of turning my holistic health–coaching practice into a much larger company that eventually became FLOliving.com. My personal need was that of expansion—not only because it was in line with my mission of serving as many women as possible, but also because as a woman it's my nature to create and expand. I couldn't help but anticipate what I wanted to do next. I had no idea if I could do it, but I wanted to try anyway. When you embrace your feminine energy as a means through which to create, you're not focused on the *endpoint*. When you commit to a life in which you spend a great deal of time in the creator role, you're being pulled by your passions and desires. You're trying new things, building in new dimensions, and letting go of what the outcome might be. That's because the creation process itself serves an innate need, and *everyone* benefits from the process—including you.

The reason why tapping into your feminine energy is the *fifth* step of the protocol and not the *first* is that when you've embarked on the first four steps, you've already observed the power your body has to change on the physical level, and this becomes easy for you to trust. You're ready, with that grounding, to take on this final piece. When you commit to your feminine energy, you give yourself the pleasure and joy of creating a healthy hormonal foundation every single day. You happily do what's required to stabilize your blood sugar, nurture your adrenals, support your pathways of elimination, and cross-train your life with your cycle, because all those things give you clear and unending access to your feminine power. That's the most profound shift you can make in all the work you've done so far. You're going to get healthy, yes, but you're also going to move into a place of extraordinary living beyond accomplishing your health goals. When you partner with your body—when you own it, care for it, and adore it—you will impregnate every single aspect of your life with its intrinsic dynamic of transformation.

Shine Like the Star You Are

I know that you still want more, because tapping into your creative energy always breeds *more* desire and creativity. Now that you've mastered the skill of improving your health by learning the language of your hormones, you feel inspired to apply your creativity even further; being a change agent is in your very biology. I know that you're feeling this way because this was my experience as well, and I watch the spark of creativity glow within my clients every single day. If someone had told me when I was eighteen that I would become an expert on women's hormonal health, open a center serving women internationally, and eventually become the CEO of a mobile healthcare company, there's no way I would've believed them. Yet my body and my hormones have led me precisely to this moment, and I know that *your* body is about to take *you* on a spectacular ride that you've only begun to imagine. I distinctly remember this feeling in my own body and mind, especially once I learned to engage my feminine energy. It's the vibration of your own potential energy—you want to channel your need to create into something purposeful and life-changing, but you may not be sure where to begin. I've got your answer right here: start with the star.

Each of the five points of the star represents a dimension of your life that gives you joy, pleasure, and fulfillment. Though the format for each star is the same (more on that below), each woman's star is nonetheless unique, because we all gain fulfillment in different ways.

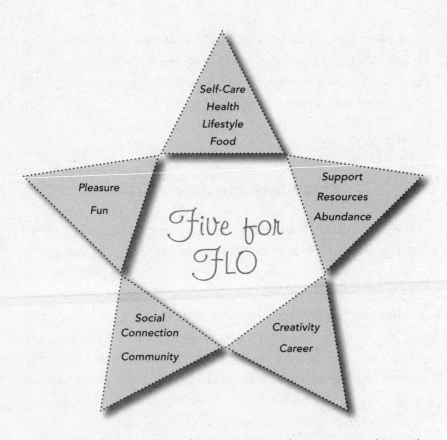

The star is like its own endocrine system: when you attend to each underlying part and support it with what it needs to thrive, you set yourself up for a happy, healthy life. Not only can you channel your inherent desire to create into attending to each of these five areas within your life; but when you feel that these five areas are working optimally, you're in the very best position to create change *outside* of yourself, too. Throughout the book you've worked to build confidence back into your connection with your body. Once you realize that you can create this transformation in your body, you will have confidence that you can transform *any* aspect of your life with the same methodical energy and dedication you applied to the WomanCode protocol.

How to Use the Star

As women, we're always looking at ways of refining how we can expand within the world around us. The star is your new framework. It contains the most essential ingredients for a healthy life plan—a plan that you can use to assess how well you're doing, one that you can keep revisiting in a cyclical fashion. When one of the points feels out of sync, spend extra time in that area, bringing it to a place where you feel centered again. Keep in mind that this exercise of examining how well you're doing should never feel like work; it should always feel like play. And, just as you trust that when you give your body the right ingredients it will take care of the rest of the healing equation, when you pour positive and constructive energy into nurturing the different areas of your life, trust that all of the right doors will open for you.

Here's what each of the five points of the star is all about:

- *Self-care, health, lifestyle, and food.* If you came to this book with hormonal imbalances, then you've already been dedicating yourself to this area through the WomanCode protocol. When this area is in balance, you're living the protocol and doing all of the things you need to do to carry it out each day, such as shopping thoughtfully for food, cooking with an eye toward health and enjoyment, making time for exercise, planning and living each month in sync with your cycle, practicing self-care, and making proactive choices that safeguard your hormonal balance.

- *Support, resources, and abundance.* This point of the star powerfully speaks to how well you're doing with engaging your feminine energy, how effectively you're using that feminine energy as a container to receive support, manage your resources, and attract wealth. It's not just about handling your finances responsibly and consciously, although that is an essential part of feeling like you're in a place where you can effortlessly create. It's also about looking at the full picture of what makes you feel abundant and how the people you rely on support you. All of these different aspects make you feel like *whatever* you want to create in your life is doable on a very fundamental level.

- *Creativity and career.* What do you care about? You know that you're actively engaged in this part of your life if you're currently dedicating yourself to whatever your answer to this question was. And when you're in this place of engagement, you feel that you're living your life with purpose. If you don't know what your career is (or should be) yet, follow your creativity and passions every week in some focused way, and that process will lead you toward a career that allows you to engage those passions every single day. Though it's not always possible to be in a career designed around your passions, it's still important to seek out activities that allow you to engage them on your own or in a group setting, such as by attending or creating conferences, classes, or organizations that serve a particular passion. This will give you value and purpose in your life no matter what your career may be.

- *Social connection and community.* At the highest level, this point of the star is about the people in your life, about surrounding yourself with those individuals who make you feel your absolute best. But it's deeper than that, too. When you're inhabiting all of the other areas of the star—when you're living in creativity and designing your career and/or life around your passions—you create beautiful interactions with like-minded people who lift you up in every possible way and value your unique gifts.

- *Pleasure and fun.* Leaving room for spontaneity, exploring new forms of pleasure, and taking risks are essential to a healthy life. Pleasure is inherently risky, but the rewards are what bring you the most joy. This area is like the fountain of youth in many ways: the more you seek out those new experiences, the more you build new neural pathways in your brain (because you're continuously learning new skills). When you dive into this area of your life, you frequently ask yourself, *Do I like . . . ?* or *Would I like . . . ?* The rest is up to your imagination: Do you like making homemade sushi? Creating pottery? Traveling? Running? Skiing? Learning French? Gardening? The drive to find out the answers to your questions will keep you continuously rebirthing pleasure in your life—and having fun along the way.

Be the Star of Your Life:
Unleash Your Organic Feminine Power

The purpose of the star is not to impel you to exist in perfect harmony within all five areas and do your best to stay there. Your life is constantly changing, and so should you be. Thus the star is about moving continuously through all these segments to continuously rebirth yourself, because that's your divine nature. It's a beautiful progression: the moment you focus your energy on one area of the star, it breathes new life into all the others, so you're always moving up and out from your starting point within the star. It's about devoting your love and attention to each of these different parts of your life so you can grow and expand in new and fulfilling ways.

If you've created a physical and emotional environment that takes into consideration all five elements of the star, you are now operating in your most potent form. When it comes to making these greater shifts in your life and in your world, you've never been in a better

SUCCESS STORY: *Daphne Blake, 44*

CONDITION: Low Libido

I started working with FLO Living in 2005. At the time I was twenty pounds overweight, I was going through a divorce, and my entire world had turned upside down. During the last eighteen months of my marriage, my husband and I rarely had sex. Finally, in my late thirties, I found the courage to leave the relationship. Part of my journey with WomanCode was to reconnect with my feminine energy as a tool to help me attract more fun, pleasure, and excitement into my life, as well as better-quality relationships. I practiced the art of setting boundaries with men whom I dated, as well as with my coworkers and family members. I went back to school to earn an MFA.

Through my work with WomanCode, I realized that my lack of libido with my ex-husband was pointing to larger underlying problems. I had some stress and health issues (such as HPV); these I dealt with quite easily using food and supplements. But the deeper issue was that I was divorced from my feminine energy. I had no idea how to be in balance with my masculine and feminine energy so that I wasn't just giving my partner what he needed, but was capable of receiving what I needed as well. Using the Principles of Feminine Energy, I rebalanced several aspects of my life—especially my career and my relationships with family and friends.

When I finally met the man of my dreams several years later, our connection was effortless, rich, and bursting with chemistry. In a FLO Living workshop I took in 2005, we had an assignment where we wrote down the qualities of our ideal man. I tried to be as honest and as specific as possible and included things like "He speaks with integrity," "He has a nice voice," and "He likes to cook." I had forgotten about that list but recently found it in a drawer. I realized, reading it so much later, that seven years to the day after I made that list, I'd married the exact man I had described. It gives me goose bumps just thinking about it. But I know that it was only through my work with WomanCode that I was able to invite this wonderful man into my life, because I had done the work on myself first.

position to connect with your internal wisdom than you are at this very moment. Now that you've removed all the FLO Blockers from your life and have balanced your hormones, you have unlimited access to your deepest desires, along with the power to create them. You're able to interpret clearly the signals that your body is sending about where it would like you to go next. It boils down to a very simple task: follow your appetite and live as a change agent. Ask yourself, *What in my life gives me the greatest sense of pleasure and purpose?* My greatest hope is that you'll use this question to create a life that is every bit as magnificent as you dreamed it would be.

One-on-One with Alisa

Masculine and Feminine Energy Balance, Principles of Feminine Energy in action, and becoming an effective creator of change—where's a gal to start? In order to best digest this all and incorporate exactly what you need in this moment to support your bigger health goals of fixing your period, improving your fertility, or recharging your libido, make a short list of what stood out for you most in this section. Following your natural interest will actually tell you a lot about where you should and can start making changes immediately. Perhaps you are intrigued by masculine and feminine energy balance during every-day situations. Are you happy with your current ratio? Experiment with a different approach (with your masculine or feminine) to see if you get a better result. If one of the principles jumped out at you, then by all means put that new mantra into action. If you are on fire and ready to make some changes beyond your physical health, then work with the star and list one clear and specific outcome you'd like to create in each area. You can come back to this chapter again and again for continuous work with step 5 of the WomanCode protocol—I do!

SUCCESS STORY: K.C. Baker, 28

CONDITION: Painful Periods, PMS, Acne

When I turned twenty-five, my health suddenly started going down the tubes. I was chronically stressed out. I lived all the time in an ever-fluctuating world of emotional turbulence. My skin was very broken out in acne. And my periods were terrible.

Eventually, a dear friend suggested I contact Alisa to see if she could help. I realized that being successful in my life was dependent upon my health, so I made the investment to do the program.

Something amazing happened during that time. Alisa helped me transform my relationship to my body. I began to really talk to my body. Food became a source of nourishment and joy instead of angst. My skin's health improved. And I began to really see where I was letting boundaries get crossed all the time in my life in various relationships. Alisa guided me in developing a very healthy and beautiful relationship with my emotions, and I am now excellent at speaking my truth in the moment when a boundary has been crossed.

Alisa taught me how to more fully nurture myself, and that impacts every area of my life. My life is richer, healthier, and more beautiful because of it, and I feel profound gratitude. I now run my own business training other women to use their voice and speak in public. I have met the love of my life and I know that the WomanCode protocol will set us up to have a healthy pregnancy when that time comes. My hope is that every woman has access to the incredibly valuable wisdom and guidance of FLO Living.

CHAPTER 10

Staying in the FLO

E very time I give a talk, lead a workshop, or connect with women in one-on-one sessions, people always ask me the same question: "Is there more?" Absolutely!

This is what I love about women and about being a woman—we are natural researchers. As the gatherers in the hunter-gatherer primitive structure, our brains are in fact hard-wired to collect resources. In the digital age, this means information. When you are confused about your body and want the *right* information *right* now, you head online and start researching. Unfortunately, when you are dealing with a health issue, there's a lot of information to wade through, some of it disheartening, some of it overly technical, and some of it untrustworthy. I'll never forget the first time I typed my condition in to a search engine—I was devastated—the prognosis was crushing and I seemed to be the only one in the world going through it. I did not yet realize that I, like so many of you, was not alone. I promised myself that if I got better, I would create that website that I wished had existed when I was first diagnosed—a place where I could get educated about my body, be trained in a natural method that would restore my health, where I could receive individual support from an expert, and where I could connect with other women going through the same thing so I would know that I was not alone. FLOliving.com is the product of that promise and my vision for a type of healthcare that we women deserve: a website and experience tailored for our unique bodies, where you can go to get all the information you need about hormones.

As you take on the WomanCode protocol, it's only natural that you will have questions you want answered specifically in regards to your body. You will want a coach who can guide you through the food changes so they stick and ensure your success. You will want a forum where you can share your experiences, WomanCode-friendly recipes, and your new commitment to hormonal health. You will crave a community that encourages you to continue growing from this new place of well-being. This book provides exactly what you need to improve your hormonal issues and play a bigger game in your life, but it's only the beginning of a lifelong adventure. That's why I launched FLOliving.com as a counterpart to this book, so you will always be able to get more information and more individual support. At FLOliving.com, you'll receive support from me, my expert FLO coaches, and women around the globe who are using the WomanCode protocol every meal, every day, and getting the results they have been after for years. I don't want to see one more woman struggle with symptoms and think to herself that it's just part of being a woman and that it's normal to not feel her best. It feels unacceptable to me that we tolerate so much dis-ease in our bodies and that there isn't a gold-standard solution out there for us.

Join the WomanCode Community

I created the book and online community as cumulative success-building pieces. When you're living this lifestyle, unexpected nuances are bound to occur in your daily life. You can access FLO expert coaches online to help you work through those personal situations. Together, the book and FLOliving.com will ensure that you're able to put every aspect of the protocol into practice every day, no matter what life throws your way. While the book provides the method, the online program and coaching give you the accountability to move more quickly into such advanced mastery that the WomanCode way is a seamless aspect of your daily life.

You may remember that one of the Principles of Feminine Energy is that women learn better collaboratively—a principle that I see proven every day. I've found that my clients are much more successful at adhering to their new lifestyle when they have people they can connect with. It's about more than exchanging information; it's about sharing a lifestyle. FLOliving.com is a virtual health center for women, and it's dedicated to supporting women's hormonal and reproductive health. We're here for you, no matter what health or lifestyle issue prompts you to seek assistance. Furthermore, though every woman comes to WomanCode with different needs, desires, and goals, we can target our help to *you* specifically: you have the opportunity to customize the degree of support you receive online and how the website works for you. Here's a glimpse of some of the resources you'll find online:

- Hormonal Sync System, our premier online program/hormonal improvement platform.

- Online video session takes you, in depth, through all five steps of the WomanCode protocol over the course of three months.

- Access to the FLO Living community, including an online question-and-answer forum where you can receive advice from our team of FLO expert coaches or other women in the FLO Living community.

- An extensive library of hormone-friendly meal suggestions, recipes, and grocery lists that support each of the four phases of your menstrual cycle.

- Regular blogs with additional resources that are relevant for your life, such as product evaluations, study highlights, guest contributors, and more.

Become a WomanCode Ambassador

I hope that, throughout this journey, you'll feel inspired to share your experience, online and in person, with the women in your life. I can't tell you how many women have said to me, "If only I'd known about WomanCode sooner, I wouldn't have spent so many years suffering needlessly." I always ask them to share this resource with the women in their lives so that other women won't have to approach me with that anguish in the future. Every woman deserves to have information and tools at her fingertips to support her right when and where she needs those tools most. I appreciate that frustration because I've been there myself. *I* was once that woman looking for answers and finding a dead end at every turn. But once I got healthy and created this protocol, it became my privilege to share what I know, and I hope you'll do the same for the women around you. There are more than twenty million women suffering from some kind of hormonal issue today. I can only begin to imagine what kind of transformation we could create together in women's healthcare if every reader like you started sharing her experience of living according to WomanCode.

I feel humbled, inspired, and motivated every time I witness a woman transform. When I receive an e-mail from a woman telling me, say, that she had her first regular menstrual cycle in three years or get pregnant finally once she started engaging the protocol, my heart swells. I'm already thinking about the incredible things this woman is going to do with her life now that she has access to her hormonal health and energetic potential. I hope you'll love the women in your life enough to share the FLO Living and WomanCode resources with them, because it's through food and a partnership with our bodies that we can heal these issues that impact every aspect of our lives. I'm deeply proud of having created this process and this platform to ensure that women all over the world have access to their birthright of healthy bodies, clear minds, and creative power. Together we can start having the right conversation about how to be healthy hormonal women.

Sourcing Your Power

Power, from the feminine energy viewpoint, is the ability to collaborate to create change. You've accessed that power to create change in your health. What I've seen that helps ensure these changes endure comes from getting involved with causes greater than yourself. Doing so keeps us motivated to be our best selves so we have the energy to be in service to that which we feel passionately about. Consider it a new form of health insurance against falling off the WomanCode protocol. By now you know I want you to be living your

Continued on page 288

purpose with your body as your foundation for success. Use this program to get healthy and live your big life—create businesses, have families, see the world, and make an impact in your communities. I want you to think big and global. As you keep living in the FLO and creating a life you love, think about how you can reach a hand out to women who don't have access to education and healthcare or rights to their bodies and the ability to earn wages. These are issues I'm totally passionate about—can you imagine a world in which all women had access to those basic freedoms? I know how critical having access to all of the above has been in allowing me to live the life of my dreams, and I dream of a world where all women are empowered to lead us into a healthier global future. By powering up your own health you can power up the lives of women around the world by helping them get access to education, create opportunities to work, and ending sexual and physical abuse. For more ways to learn about these issues and how you can help, connect with the Half the Sky movement on their website.

Together we can usher in a new global feminine paradigm with health and opportunity for all women. We are all connected by our unique and dynamic biochemistry. Take care of your body and help women worldwide take better care of themselves.

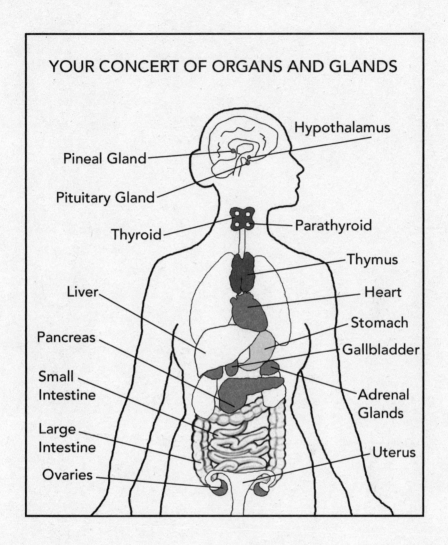

YOUR CONCERT OF ORGANS AND GLANDS

Hypothalamus

Pineal Gland

Pituitary Gland

Thyroid — Parathyroid

Thymus

Liver — Heart

Pancreas — Stomach

Gallbladder

Small Intestine

Adrenal Glands

Large Intestine

Uterus

Ovaries

ALISA'S
MEDICINE CABINET

My personal medicine cabinet—and the one I recommend for all women creating a symptom-free future—is packed with supplements, spices, herbs, and teas. The most important thing to keep in mind when it comes to supplements is that they're exactly that—supplements to, not substitutes for, a healthy diet. When used appropriately, they can be a powerful aid in short-term healing. If you're currently engaged in the WomanCode protocol and are changing the foods that you eat, this is an ideal time to use supplements to help expedite the process of improving your endocrine function.

Here's how to use the list below. You'll notice that the supplements, many of which have been discussed in the main text, are grouped into categories. As you're focusing on each part of the protocol, focus on using supplements from the relevant group. When you move on to the next step, transition to choosing supplements from that step of the protocol.

It's important to take occasional breaks from supplements. Every three to four months stop using them entirely. This break can be a wonderful way to gauge how your body is doing on its own and can help inform you about the ways the supplements are helping you. If you don't notice a difference when you stop taking them, your body may be doing a beautiful job on its own; in that case, you no longer need the support of those supplements.

Finally, a crucial part of maintaining a healthy medicine cabinet is proper storage. Be sure to keep your supplements, herbs, spices, and teas away from heat, moisture, and light, elements that break down the compounds in your supplements and make them less effective (or alter the way that they work entirely). So keep those items out of the bathroom and away from the sink and stove in the kitchen. For more guidance on usage or dosage, or if you have specific questions about which supplements are best for you, visit FLOliving.com to speak with a FLO expert coach.*

For Blood Sugar Stability

- Cinnamon
- Chromium picolinate
- Tea with rooibos, cinnamon, anise, and/or peppermint (drink after a meal)

For Adrenal Health

- To support mental focus—ginkgo biloba, rhodiola
- To increase energy—ashwagandha, vitamin B12, vitamin B5
- To reduce stress—holy basil (use in tea)

---

* Doses will vary based on product. Follow general dosing instructions on packaging, or contact us.

- To get off caffeine but feel like you're drinking black tea/coffee—kukicha, also known as twig tea (made from the stem, later roasted, from which green tea leaves have been plucked)

For Improved Elimination

- Large intestine—organic ground flaxseed, oat bran, acacia (fibers); *Saccharomyces boulardii* and *Lactobacillus rhamnosus* (probiotics). Store the flaxseed in the refrigerator or freezer in a resealable bag, squeezing air out each time to prevent oxidation, which can decrease the fiber and omega-3 content. Rotate the above-named fibers, using one source of fiber daily for two weeks at a time.

- Liver—B-100 complex (containing all the B vitamins at 100 percent of the recommended daily allowance or greater), inositol, artichoke leaf (supports the thyroid too), burdock tea, Get Clean tea by Republic of Tea (containing, among other things, milk thistle, burdock, and dandelion)

For Cycle Support

- Vitex capsules
- Magnesium-calcium blend (in ionic powdered form)
- Tea with dong quai for the first half of the cycle (Yogi Tea's Women's Energy)
- Tea containing raspberry leaf, nettle, and parsley leaf (to help with bloating and with flushing built-up fluids) for the second half of the cycle

For Immune-Strengthening and Anti-Inflammatory Effects

- L-glutamine, n-acetyl-l-glucosamine, quercetin
- Green "Superfood" powder, any type containing organic veggies, berries, wheatgrass, spirulina
- Chlorella tablets—they bond with heavy metals in the body and pull them out through your bowels
- Turmeric supplement with active curcumin
- Omega-3 purified fish-oil capsules
- Vitamin C-ester tablets with citrus-based bioflavonoids
- Zinc tablets
- Black elderberry extract—great for when you're sick with a cold or flu
- Apple cider vinegar

WOMANCODE-APPROVED PRODUCTS

Body Complaint	Product Remedies	Why I Love Them
Skin breakouts	John Masters's Oily Skin Serum	This serum contains aloe and bacteria-eating probiotics to stop breakouts and soothe inflamed skin.
	Earth Science's A/B Hydroxy Repair	It's gentle enough to use every other night to turn over skin cells and prevent clogged pores from forming.
Bloating	Rainbow Light's EnzyMend Digestive Aid	It contains all-natural plant-based enzymes and therapeutic herbs to aid digestion and soothe intestines, thereby preventing bloating.
	Herb Pharm Fennel tincture	Try this potent tincture, or just the vegetable itself, which is a natural digestive aid and bloat-reducer.

Body Complaint	Product Remedies	Why I Love Them
Urinary tract infection	Source Naturals' D-Mannose	Derived from a nutrient found in fruit, this supplement is a more effective alternative to cranberry juice that won't overload your blood sugar levels. Prevents bacteria from adhering to lining of bladder.
Yeast infection	Yeast Arrest's Vitanica Suppositories	The best natural remedy I've found for stubborn yeast infections.
Fatigue/foggy-headedness	Jarrow Formulas' Adrenal Optimizer New Chapter's Rhodiola	Contains vitamins and herbs that nourish and boost your adrenal gland function. Dating back to the ancient Greeks, this herb is a powerful stress reliever, immune booster, and energy/mental-focus enhancer.
	Eden's Organic Kukicha Twig Tea	Roasted, robust flavor and gentle, moderate caffeine levels make this tea a great alternative to coffee that will keep you alert without burning you out.
Constipation	ReNew Life's FiberSMART	Taken daily, this combo of flax, probiotics, and intestine-lubricating herbs is a great way to keep things moving. Regular bowel movements are key in hormonal balance!
Low blood sugar	Pure Bar Organic	These bars are easily transportable and packed with only simple, whole foods. Always keep an emergency stash in your purse! Bonus: they're gluten-free and come in yummy flavors.

MEDICINAL FOODS FOR HORMONAL SYMPTOMS

As you eat healthy, natural foods that support hormone balance and as you learn to honor and respect the needs of your cycle, you may still continue to experience certain symptoms. These symptoms are messages from your body letting you know that your organ system needs tuning. When this occurs, refer to the dietary adjustments below, which are particularly helpful and healing for each of the following symptoms:

Acne/Pimples/Blackheads

- *Increase water*
- *Increase leafy greens*
- *Reduce processed foods*
- *Reduce sugar*
- *Reduce animal protein*

Anovulation

- *Increase warm water*
- *Increase root vegetables*
- *Increase beans/tofu*
- *Increase sea vegetables*
- *Reduce sugar*
- *Reduce dairy*

Bleeding: Heavy

- *Increase water with lemon*
- *Increase leafy greens*
- *Reduce animal protein*
- *Reduce spicy food*

Bleeding: Light/Stagnant

- *Increase warm water*
- *Increase root vegetables*
- *Increase beans*
- *Increase sea vegetables*
- *Increase healthy oils*
- *Reduce animal protein*

Bloating

- *Increase water*
- *Increase fennel*
- *Increase leafy greens*
- *Reduce salt*
- *Reduce processed foods*

Breast Pain or Tenderness

- *Increase fennel*
- *Increase leafy greens*
- *Increase water*
- *Reduce dairy*
- *Reduce caffeine*

Constipation

- *Increase water*
- *Increase fruit*
- *Increase sweet potatoes*
- *Increase leafy greens*
- *Reduce processed foods*

Fatigue

- *Increase water*
- *Increase sea vegetables*
- *Increase healthy protein*
- *Reduce sugar*
- *Reduce caffeine*

Irritability

- *Increase leafy greens*
- *Increase whole grains*
- *Increase chocolate*
- *Reduce animal protein*
- *Reduce dairy*
- *Reduce caffeine*

Low Libido

- *Increase sea vegetables*
- *Increase beans*
- *Increase root vegetables*
- *Increase water*
- *Increase spicy foods*
- *Increase chocolate*
- *Reduce alcohol*

Mood Swings and Sugar Lows

- *Increase sweet veggies*
- *Increase whole grains*
- *Increase green drinks*
- *Increase water*
- *Increase healthy protein*
- *Reduce sugar*
- *Reduce caffeine*

Pelvic Pain/Cramping

- *Increase water*
- *Reduce protein*
- *Reduce caffeine*
- *Reduce alcohol*

Urinary Tract Infection

- *Increase water*
- *Increase cranberry tea*
- *Increase greens*
- *Increase beans/tofu*
- *Increase sea vegetables*
- *Reduce animal protein*

Yeast Infection

- *Increase garlic and onion*
- *Increase millet*
- *Increase spicy foods*
- *Reduce cold and raw foods*
- *Reduce soy products*
- *Reduce foods with yeast*

BIBLIOGRAPHY

Abravanel, Elliot D., Elizabeth A. King and Alan Sandborne. *Dr. Abravanel's Body Type Diet and Lifetime Nutrition Plan*. New York: Bantam, 1999.

Agus, David B. *The End of Illness*. New York: Simon & Schuster Ltd, 2012.

Aihara, Herman. *Acid and Alkaline*. California: George Ohsawa Macrobiotic, 1986.

Angier, Natalie. *Woman: An Intimate Geography*. Massachusetts: Houghton Mifflin Harcourt, 1999.

Balch, Phyllis A., and James F. *Prescription for Nutritional Healing*. New York: Avery Publishing, 1990.

Behan, Eileen. *Therapeutic Nutrition: A Guide to Patient Education*. Pennsylvania: Lippincott Williams & Wilkins, 2005.

Beinfield, Harriet and Efram Korngold. *Between Heaven and Earth: A Guide to Chinese Medicine*. New York: Ballantine Books, 1991.

Bodansky, Steve Ph.D., and Vera Bodansky Ph.D. *The Illustrated Guide to Extended Massive Orgasm*. California: Hunter House, 2002.

Brizendine, Louann. *The Female Brain*. New York: Three Rivers Press, 2007.

Colbin, Annemarie. *Food and Healing*. New York: Ballantine Books, 1996.

David, Marc. *Nourishing Wisdom: A Mind-Body Approach to Nutrition and Well-Being*. New York: Three Rivers Press, 1994.

Dean, Carolyn. *Hormone Balance: A Woman's Guide To Restoring Health And Vitality*. New York: Adams Media, 2005.

Domar, Alice, and Henry Dreher. *Healing Mind, Healthy Woman: Using the Mind-Body Connection to Manage Stress and Take Control of Your Life*. New York: Delta, 1997.

Erasmus, Udo. *Fats That Heal, Fats That Kill: The Complete Guide to Fats, Oils, Cholesterol and Human Health*. Canada: Alive Books, 1993.

Fallon, Sally, and Mary Enig. *Nourishing Traditions: The Cookbook that Challenges Politically Correct Nutrition and the Diet Dictocrats*. Indiana: Newtrends Publishing, Inc., 1999. (revised & updated 2nd edition)

Gates, Donna, and Linda Schatz. *The Body Ecology Diet: Recovering Your Health and Rebuilding Your Immunity*. California: Body Ecology, 1996.

Groll, Jeremy. *Fertility Foods: Optimize Ovulation and Conception Through Food Choices* Canada: Fireside, 2006.

Hadady, Letha. *Asian Health Secrets: The Complete Guide to Asian Herbal Medicine*. New York: Three Rivers Press, 1998. (1st edition)

Harris, Colette, and Theresa Cheung. *PCOS Diet Book: How You Can Use the Nutritional Approach to Deal with Polycystic Ovary Syndrome*. New York: Thorsons, 2002.

Hay, Louise. *Heal Your Body*. California: Hay House, 1984.

Lu, Henry C. *Chinese Natural Cures*. New York: Black Dog & Leventhal, 1994. (1st edition)

Hudson, Tori. *Women's Encyclopedia of Natural Medicine: Alternative Therapies and Integrative Medicine for Total Health and Wellness*. New York: McGraw-Hill, 2007. (2nd edition)

Kapit, Wynn. *The Anatomy Coloring Book*. California: Benjamin Cummings, 2001. (3rd edition)

Kapit, Wynn, Robert I. Macey, and Esmail Meisami. Kapit. *The Physiology Coloring Book*. California: Benjamin Cummings, 1999. (2nd edition)

Kaptchuk, Ted. *The Web That Has No Weaver : Understanding Chinese Medicine*. New York: McGraw-Hill, 2000. (2nd edition)

Katz, David L. *Nutrition in Clinical Practice: A Comprehensive, Evidence-Based Manual for the Practitioner , 2nd Edition*. Pennsylvania: Lippincott Williams & Wilkins, 2008.

Kloss, Jethro. *Back to Eden*. Wisconsin: Lotus Press, 2005.

Lee, John R., and Virginia Hopkins. *Dr. John Lee's Hormone Balance Made Simple: The Essential How-to Guide to Symptoms, Dosage, Timing, and More*. New York: Grand Central Life & Style, 2006.

Lipski, Elizabeth. *Digestive Wellness: Strengthen the Immune System and Prevent Disease Through Healthy Digestion*. McGraw-Hill: New York, 2005. (3rd edition)

Martin, Raquel, Judi Gerstung, and John Hart. *The Estrogen Alternative: A Guide to Natural Hormonal Balance*. Vermont: Healing Arts Press, 2004. (4th edition)

Tiwari, Maya. *Women's Power to Heal: Through Inner Medicine*. Pennsylvania: Mother Om Media, 2012.

Muir, Charles, and Caroline Muir. Tantra: *The Art of Conscious Loving*. California: Mercury House, 1989.

Murray, Michael T., Joseph Pizzorno, and Lara Pizzorno. *The Encyclopedia of Healing Foods*. New York: Atria Books, 2005. (1st edition)

Northrup, Christiane. *Women's Bodies, Women's Wisdom: Creating Physical and Emotional Health and Healing*. New York: Bantam, 2010. (revised edition)

Pitchford, Paul. *Healing with Whole Foods: Asian Traditions and Modern Nutrition*. California: North Atlantic Books, 2003. (3rd edition)

Murray, Michael T., and Joseph Pizzorno. *The Encyclopedia of Natural Medicine Third Edition*. New York: Atria Books, 2012.

Schulz, Mona Lisa. *The New Feminine Brain: Developing Your Intuitive Genius*. New York: Free Press, 2006.

Sher, Geoffrey, Virginia Marriage Davis, and Jean Stoess. *In Vitro Fertilization: The A.R.T of Making Babies*. New York: Facts on File, 2005. (3rd edition)

Steelsmith, Laurie, and Alex Steelsmith. *Natural Choices for Women's Health: How the Secrets of Natural and Chinese Medicine Can Create a Lifetime of Wellness*. New York: Three Rivers Press, 2005.

Tiwari, Maya. *Ayurveda: A Life of Balance: The Complete Guide to Ayurvedic Nutrition & Body Types with Recipes*. Vermont: Healing Arts Press, 1994. (1st edition)

Thomashauer, Regena. *Mama Gena's School of Womanly Arts : Using the Power of Pleasure to Have Your Way with the World*. New York: Simon & Schuster, 2003.

Turner, Natasha. *The Hormone Diet: A 3-Step Program to Help You Lose Weight, Gain Strength, and Live Younger Longer*. Pennsylvania: Rodale Books, 2011. (1 Int Edition)

Reiss, Uzzi, and Martin Zucker. *Natural Hormone Balance for Women: Look Younger, Feel Stronger, and Live Life with Exuberance*. New York: Atria Books, 2002.

Vliet, Elizabeth Lee. *It's My Ovaries Stupid!*. New York: Scribner, 2003.

Weed, Susun S. *New Menopausal Years : The Wise Woman Way, Alternative Approaches for Women 30-90*. New York: Ash Tree Publishing, 2002. (revised edition)

Weschler, Toni. *Taking Charge of Your Fertility, 10th Anniversary Edition: The Definitive Guide to Natural Birth Control, Pregnancy Achievement, and Reproductive Health*. New York: Quill Press, 2002.

ACKNOWLEDGMENTS

My family: To my mother who has unconditionally supported all my desires to get healthy naturally, to follow my unusual career choice after Hopkins, and for lovingly and selflessly making the home from which my body, my heart, and my spirit could soar. To my father who first nurtured me to be the bold, independent, and curious woman I am today.

To my two grandmothers on whose powerful shoulders I stand. To my brothers and my sisters-in-law, and the beautiful children they have brought into my life—my family is a joy. To Jelena Petrovic who is my soul sister, separated at birth, reunited at Hopkins—I love you beyond measure and am so grateful for our many sushi dinners toasting to each other's dreams. To my cousin Lori Feeney for the most hilarious phone chats that keep me grounded.

My company: To my amazing team at FLOliving.com—Brandi Hand for writing that letter that started our working relationship, all of your social media genius, and for your friendship; Stefanie Torrieri for taking such amazing care of our community and for coming back to FLO after finishing your MBA; Jessica Grippo—sister—for being there during every stage of growth internal and external; Jen, Carol, Shannon, Christina, Jennie, Teri—all the counselors—you are my family. Enormous gratitude to our "angels" who back the vision and mission of FLOliving.com. Special thanks to Shazi Visram for encouraging me to think bigger.

All of my clients: Your desire to find your true health and your life's passion drives me to serve. I am so lucky that I get to work with you all. And to all the doctors who have referred and keep referring women to FLO Living—you are ahead of your time.

My community: To my childhood next-door-neighbor Janice, whose two children I babysat regularly and who had three books at her home that I read around the age of twelve that would only be the beginning: *The Joy of Sex, What to Expect When You're Expecting,* and *Diet for a Small Planet.* To Britt Bursell and Lauren Sudeall—my oldest friends and constant cheerleaders. To Meggan Watterson, LiYana Silver, and K.C. Baker for being committed to the fierce feminine within and always holding up the mirror for me with love. To my amazing colleagues and friends who keep inspiring me: Kris Carr, Mastin Kipp, Gabby Bernstein, Ophira Edut, Melanie Notkin, Kate Northrup, Sabina Ptacin—you rock.

My book: To the wonderful and musical Ned Leavitt who is the most amazing literary agent ever for women's issues, and for his amazing heart-centered negotiating that gets it more than done. I'm honored to be in the company of your other clients.

Nancy Hancock at Harper, I will be ever grateful for your fierce passion to bring me and my first book into the world. You are a totally brilliant editor.

Patty Gift at Hay House for being a friend and ally.

Cheryl Richardson and Reid Tracy for selecting my video out of the thousands submitted that made me the very first Hay House mover & shaker and for giving me the opportunity to speak at the Hay House conferences.

Dr. Northrup for your giant ovaries, for courageously breaking ground with *Women's Bodies, Women's Wisdom,* for including me in WBWW, for the tarot card reading at your kitchen table where you decided it was time for me to write this book, for the countless e-mails of encouragement, and for passing me the torch.

My love: To my husband Victor Russo—for believing in this book and my vision on our very first date long before I ever had a book deal and for being the most extraordinary person with whom I get to share my life.

NOTES

Page 31. Popat, Vaishali B, Tamara Prodanov, Karim A. Calis, Lawrence M. Nelson. "The Menstrual Cycle: A Biological Marker of General Health in Adolescents." *Annals of The New York Academy of Sciences* 1135 (2008): 43–51. doi:10.1196/annals.1429.040.

Page 35. Kidd, Karen A., Paul J. Blanchfield, Kenneth H. Mills, Vince P. Palace, Robert E. Evans, James M. Lazorchake, and Robert W. Flick. "Collapse of a Fish Population After Exposure to a Synthetic Estrogen." *Proceedings of the National Academy of Sciences of the United States of America* 104 (2007): 8897–8901. doi:10.1073/pnas.0609568104.

Page 36. Smith-Spangler, Crystal, Margaret L. Brandeau, Grace E. Hunter, J. Clay Bavinger, Maren Pearson, Paul J. Eschbach, Vandana Sundaram, Hau Liu, Patricia Schirmer, Christopher Stave, Inram Olkin, Dena M. Bravata. "Are Organic Foods Safer or Healthier Than Conventional Alternatives?" *Annals of Internal Medicine* 157 (2012): 348–366.

Page 38. Stokes, Paul. "Body Absorbs 5 lb. of Make-up Chemicals a Year." The Telegraph, Jun 21, 2007. http://www.telegraph.co.uk/news/uknews/1555173/Body-absorbs–5lb-of-make-up-chemicals-a-year.html.

Page 40. Jiménez-Chillaron, Josep C., Rubén Díaz, Débora Martínez, Thais Pentinat, Marta Ramón-Krauel, Sílvia Ribó, Torsten Plösch. "The Role of Nutrition on Epigenetic Modifications and Their Implications on Health." *Biochimie* 94 (2012): 2242–2263. doi.org/10.1016/j.biochi.2012.06.012.

Page 40. Niculescu, Mihai D., Daniel S. Lupu, and Corneliu N. Craciunescu. "Perinatal Manipulation of a-Linolenic Acid Intake Induces Epigenetic Changes in Maternal and Offspring Livers." *FASEB Journal* 26 (2012). doi:10.1096/fj.12–210724.

Page 40. Pentinat, Thais, Marta Ramón-Krauel, Judith Cebria, Rubén Diaz, Josep C. Jiménez-Chillaron. "Transgenerational Inheritance of Glucose Intolerance in a Mouse Model of Neonatal Overnutrition." *Endocrinology* 151 (2010): 5617–5623. doi:10.1210/en.2010–0684.

Page 40. Nedeltcheva, Arlet V., Jennifer M. Kikus, Jacqueline Imperial, Dale A. Schoeller, Plamen D. Penev. "Insufficient Sleep Undermines Dietary Efforts to Reduce Adiposity." *Annals of Internal Medicine* 153 (2010): 435–441. doi:10.1059/0003–4819–153–7–201010050–00006.

Page 41. Spalding, Kirsty L., Ratan D. Bhardwaj, Bruce A. Buchholz, Henrik Druid, Jonas Frisen. "Retrospective Birth Dating of Cells in Humans." *Cell* 122 (2005): 133–143. doi:10.1016/j.cell.2005.04.028.

Page 44. Balbi, Carlo, Rosalia Musone, Agostino Menditto, Luigi Di Prisco, Eufemia Cassese, Maurizio D'Ajello, Domenico Ambrosio, Antonio Cardone. "Influence of Menstrual Factors and Dietary Habits on Menstrual Pain in Adolescence Age." *Gynecology and Reproductive Biology* 91 (2000): 143–148. doi:10.1016/S0301–2115(99)00277–8.

Page 46. Quaas, Alexander, and Anuja Dokras. "Diagnosis and Treatment of Unexplained Infertility." *Reviews in Obstetrics & Gynecology* 2 (2008): 69–76.

Page 49. Linos, Eleni, Walter C. Willett, Eunyoung Cho, Graham Colditz, Lindsay A. Frazier. "Red Meat Consumption during Adolescence among Premenopausal Women and Risk of Breast Cancer." *Cancer Epidemiology, Biomarkers & Prevention* 17 (2008): 2146–2151.

Page 49. Vom Saal, Frederick S. "Could Hormone Residues Be Involved?" *Human Reproduction* 22 (2007): 150–1505. doi:10.1093/humrep/dem092.

Page 49. Offer, Shira, and Barbara Schneider. "Revisiting the Gender Gap in Time-Use Patterns: Multitasking and Well-Being among Mothers and Fathers in Dual-Earner Families." *American Sociological Review* 76 (2011): 809–899. doi:10.1177/0003122411425170.

Page 80. Jones, Rachel K. "Beyond Birth Control: The Overlooked Benefits of Oral Contraceptive Pills." Guttmacher Institute, 2011. http://www.guttmacher.org/pubs/Beyond-Birth-Control.pdf.

Page 82. Roberts, S. Craig, L. Morris Gosling, Vaughan Carter, Marion Petrie. "MHC-correlated Odour Preferences in Humans and the Use of Oral Contraceptives." *Proceedings of the Royal Society B* 275 (2008): 2715–2722. doi:10.1098/rspb.2008.0825 1471–2954.

Page 89. Page, Kathleen A., Dongju Seo, Renata Belfort-DeAguiar, Cheryl Lacadie, James Dzuira, Sarita Naik, Suma Amarnath, R. Todd Constable, Robert S. Sherwin, Rajita Sinha. "Circulating Glucose Levels Modulate Neural Control of Desire for High-Calorie Foods in Humans." *Journal of Clinical Investigation* 121 (2011): 4161–4169. doi:10.1172/JCI57873.

Page 92. Levitzky, Yamini S., Michael J. Pencina, Ralph B. D'Agostino, James B. Meigs, Joanne Murabito, Ramachandran S. Vasan, Caroline S. Fox. "Impact of Impaired Fasting Glucose on Cardiovascular Disease: The Framingham Heart Study." *Journal of the American College of Cardiology* 51 (2008): 264–270.

Page 149. Durante, Kristina M., Vladas Griskevicius, Sarah E. Hill, Carin Perilloux, Norman P. Li. "Ovulation, Female Competition, and Product Choice: Hormonal Influences on Consumer Behavior." *Journal of Consumer Research* 37 (2011): 921–934.

Page 166. Brasil, F. B., Soares, L. L. , Faria, T. S., Noaventura, G. T., Sampaio, F. J. Urogenital Research Unit, State University of Rio de Janeiro, Rio de Janeiro, Brazil. *Anat Rec* (Hoboken). 2009 Apr;292(4):587-94. doi: 10.1002/ar.20878.

Page 166. Doerge, D. R., Sheehan, D. M. "Goitrogenic and Astrogenic Activity of Soy Isoflavones." Division of Biochemical Toxicology, National Center for Toxicological Research, Jefferson, Arkansas, USA. *Environ Health Perspect.* 2002 Jun;110 Suppl 3:349–53.

Page 169. Zaidi, Zeenat F. "Gender Differences in Human Brain: A Review." *Open Anatomy Journal* 2 (2010): 37–55.

Page 177. Kober, Hedy, Peter Mende-Siedlecki, Ethan F. Kross, Jochen Weber, Walter Mischel, Carl L. Hart, Kevin N. Ochsner. "Prefrontal-striatal Pathway Underlies Cognitive Regulation of Craving." *Proceedings of the National Academy of Sciences of the United States of America* 107 (2010): 14811–14816. doi:10.1073/pnas.1007779107.

Page 186. Floresco, Stan B. "Neural Circuits Underlying Behavioral Flexibility." *American Psychological Association* (2011). http://www.apa.org/science/about/psa/2011/04/neural-circuits.aspx.

Page 205. "Fertility, Family Planning, and Reproductive Health of U.S. Women: Data from the 2002 National Survey of Family Growth." U.S. Department of Health and Human Services (2005). http://www.cdc.gov/nchs/data/series/sr_23/sr23_025.pdf.

Page 205. "What Is Assisted Reproductive Technology?" Centers for Disease Control and Prevention. http://www.cdc.gov/art/.

Page 213. Colaci, D. S., M. Afeiche, A. J. Gaskins, D. R. Wright, T. L. Toth, R. Hauser, J. E. Chavarro. "Dietary Fat Intake and In-Vitro Fertilization Outcomes: Saturated Fat Intake Is Associated with Fewer Metaphase 2 Oocytes." *Human Reproduction* 27 (2012): ii78–ii79. doi:10.1093/humrep/27.s2.52.

Page 213. Cheungsamarn, Somlak, Suthee Rattanamongkolgul, Rataya Luechapudiporn, Chada Phisalaphong, Siwanon Jirawatnotai. "Curcumin Extract for Prevention of Type 2 Diabetes." *Diabetes Care* (2012). doi:10.2337/dc12–0116.

Page 213. Colaci, D. S., M. Afeiche, A. J. Gaskins, D. R. Wright, T. L. Toth, R. Hauser, J. E. Chavarro. "Dietary Fat Intake and In-Vitro Fertilization Outcomes: Saturated Fat Intake Is Associated with Fewer Metaphase 2 Oocytes." *Human Reproduction* 27 (2012): ii78–ii79. doi:10.1093/humrep/27.s2.52.

Page 215. Kesmodel, U. S., M. W. Cristensen, B. Degn, H. J. Ingerslev. "Does Coffee Consumption Reduce the Chance of Pregnancy and Live Birth in IVF." *Human Reproduction* 27 (2012): ii78–ii79. doi:10.1093/humrep/27.s2.52.

Page 215. Wright, Victoria Clay, Laura A. Schieve, Meredith A. Reynolds, Gary Jeng. "Assisted Reproductive Technology Surveillance—United States, 2002." National Center for Chronic Disease Prevention and Health Promotion, Division of Reproductive Health (2005). http://www.cdc.gov/mmwr/preview/mmwrhtml/ss5402a1.htm.

Page 220. "Women Matter." McKinsey & Company (2007). http://www.mckinsey.com/locations/paris/home/womenmatter/pdfs/Women_matter_oct2007_english.pdf.

Page 221. Wooley, Anita, and Thomas Malone. "Defend Your Research: What Makes a Team Smarter? More Women." *Harvard Business Review* (2011). http://hbr.org/2011/06/defend-your-research-what-makes-a-team-smarter-more-women/ar/1.

Page 224. "Pelvic Inflammatory Disease." Centers for Disease Control and Prevention. http://www.cdc.gov/std/pid/stdfact-pid.htm

Page 226. Hart, Roger, Dorota A. Doherty, Ian A. Newman, Craig E. Pennell, John P. Newham. "Periodontal Disease—A Further Potentially Modifiable Risk Factor Limiting Conception—A Case for a Pre-pregnancy Dental Check-up?" *Human Reproduction* 26 (2011): i70.

Page 234. Chivers, Meredith L., and J. Michael Bailey. "A Sex Difference in Features That Elicit Genital Response." *Biological Psychology* 70 (2005): 115–120.

Page 235. Masters, William H., and Virginia E. Johnson. *Human Sexual Response.* New York, Isihi Press International: 1966.

Page 244. Weeks, David, and Jamie James. *Secrets of the Superyoung: The Scientific Reasons Some People Look Ten Years Younger Than They Really Are—and How You Can, Too.* New York, Berkley: 1999.

Page 254. Panzer, C., S. Wise, G. Fantini, D. Kang, R. Munarriz, A. Guay, I. Goldstein. "Impact of Oral Contraceptives on Sex Hormone-binding Globulin and Androgen Levels: A Retrospective Study in Women with Sexual Dysfunction." *Journal of Sexual Medicine* 3 (2006): 104–113.

INDEX

Accutane, 16
acne/rosacea/eczema, 1, 3, 43, 53, 99, 108, 175, 282, 295, 297
ACTH (adrenocorticotropic hormone), 65–66, 100
acupuncture, 28, 221
adrenal fatigue: challenging condition of, 3, 59; description of, 99–100; elevated estrogen levels due to, 80; how to exercise with, 102–3; Kathryn Hiller's success in reducing, 72; Naomi Kent's success in overcoming, 95; silent epidemic of, 1; symptoms of, 53, 174–75. *See also* libido; nurture your adrenals
adrenal glands: Alisa's medicine cabinet for health of, 292–93; cortex of the, 100–101; foods that nurture the, 249; HPA (hypothalamic-pituitary-adrenal) axis, 35, 65–66, 100, 212, 219; medulla of the, 101–3; mismanaged blood sugar as stressor for, 81–83, 98–99. *See also* stress
adrenals, 60
adrenocorticotropic hormone (ACTH), 63
airport security, 226
alcohol consumption, 43, 183–84, 189–91, 298
Aldactone, 16
aldosterone, 101
Alisa's medicine cabinet: for adrenal health, 292–93; for blood sugar stability, 292; for cycle support, 293; for immune-strengthening and anti-inflammatory effects, 294; for improved elimination, 293; recommendations from, 291–92. *See also* supplements

allergies: gluten sensitivity, 196–97, 199; as hormonal imbalance symptom, 113, 175
Alzheimer's disease, 73
amenorrhea, 3
American Association of Drugless Practitioners, 22
anti-inflammatory products, 294
anxiety: adrenal fatigue and, 100; Naomi Kent's success in overcoming, 95; as symptom of hormonal imbalance, 43; toxic lifestyle and chronic low-grade, 35; WomanCode protocol to improve, 27
applied kinesiology, 30
arousal (excitement phase), 235
avocados, 218

Baker, K.C., 282
barrier birth control methods, 86–87
Basic Brown Rice Recipe, 122
beans/legumes, 159, 298, 299
beauty products, 38–39
Be in the Know: FLO, 42; WomanCode, 42
biofeedback, 62
birth control: the Pill used for, 14, 16, 81, 82–85, 168–69, 224, 254; WomanCode recommended methods of, 86–87
bisphenol A (BPA), 35
Blake, Daphne, 280
bleeding: medicinal foods to help with heavy or light/stagnant, 298; "Seeing Red" to interpret your, 154, 208
bloating, 175, 195, 295, 298
blood pressure medication, 16
blood sugar: endocrine system cues sent through, 59, 78–83, 98–99, 174; heart disease connection to, 73, 93–94;

blood sugar, *continued*
hypoglycemia (low blood sugar), 90–92, 96, 105, 174; WomanCode Zone 1: pancreas and liver controlling, 64–65. *See also* glucose
blood sugar management: Alisa's medicine cabinet for, 292; "every meal, every day" approach to, 89; Four Day Reset of WomanCode for, 114–40; heart disease prevention through, 93–94; tips for all-day, 96–98; WomanCode-approved products for, 295; WomanCode protocol for stabilizing your, 59, 86–98, 114–40
blood sugar mismanagement: fertility issues due to, 80–81; hormonal problems due to, 59; low libido due to, 81–83, 98–99; menstrual problems linked to, 79–80
blue/black foods, 249
body: checks and balances of body chemistry of the, 45–46; the endocrine system of your, 3–6, 44–46; during four phases of menstrual cycle, 146, 148, 150, 152; mind-body connection, 62; rebuilding your relationship with your, 167–70; Traditional Chinese Medicine (TCM) as framework for understanding your, 19, 107, 249; WomanCode-approved products for complaints of the, 295–96. *See also* brain
Bohannon, Emily, 158
Bok Choy Salad, 120
bowel movements, 110–11, 139
brain: gender differences of women's and men's, 169; HPA (hypothalamic-pituitary-adrenal) axis of the, 35, 65–66, 100, 212, 219; HPO (hypothalamic-pituitary-ovarian) axis of the, 69; during the menstrual phase, 152–53; mind-body connection and the, 62; neurotransmitters in the, 238; prefrontal cortex of the, 91, 177–78; reward system of the, 177; sexual responses and role of your, 237–41. *See also* body
Braun, Heidi, 201
breakfasts/early morning snacks: Four Day Reset, 126, 129, 132, 136–37; for syncing your cycle, 162, 163
breasts: fibrocystic, 32, 43, 46; hormone-sensitivity of, 68; as "lady parts," 60; medicinal foods to treat pain or tenderness, 298; tender, 46
buckwheat, 217
busy work-time, 187–89

caffeine, 96, 100, 214–15, 248, 293, 299
calcium supplement, 227

CAM (complementary and alternative medicine) therapies: acupuncture, 28, 221; applied kinesiology, 30; chiropractic treatment, 30; health benefits of, 28; herbalism, 30; massage, 29, 221; naturopathy, 29
cancer, 73, 85
caraway seeds, 115
carbs: comparing fast versus slow burners' need for, 93; craving/binging on, 43, 91–92, 177; during holidays and family-time events, 191–94; hypoglycemia beginning with overindulging in, 90–92, 96, 105; managing late-night overload on, 184–85; managing your blood sugar all day by limiting, 96–98. *See also* foods
career: demands of work and, 187–89; masculine/feminine balance in your life and, 263–67; star dimension on creativity and, 276, 278; taking vacations from work, 271–72
chickpeas, 217
Chinese royal physician, 107
chiropractic treatment, 30
chocolate: as blue/black food, 249; craving, 43, 61; eating, 190, 194, 298; ovulatory phase and eating, 160
cholesterol levels, 94
chronic BV (bacterial vaginosis), 209
chronic respiratory infections, 53
chronic sinusitis, 113
chronobiology, 19, 20
cinnamon, 218
circadian rhythms, 101, 104
cleanse enhancer recipes, 125
Clean Sweep assignments, 128, 131, 134–35
clitoris, 60
Clomid, 16, 223
coffee, 100, 214–15, 248
cold hands, 53
Collards, 122
colonics, 111
Columbia University's Teachers College, 21
conception. *See* fertility optimization
condom use, 85, 86, 87, 224, 225
constipation, 108, 110–11, 139, 175, 296, 298
corpus luteum, 150
cortisol, 99, 101, 102, 103, 239–40
creative lives, 219–22, 278
cross-training: cycle syncing as, 143–70, 171–73, 241–44; as part of the dynamic equation, 172; of your life with your hormones, 171–72
cultural conditioning, 34–35
curcumin, 216

cystic ovaries: challenging condition of, 3; as symptom of hormonal imbalance, 43

Daily WomanCode Survival Kit, 181–86
dairy foods, 196–98, 298
Decode Your Hormonal Clues. *See* endocrine system clues
dental health/flossing, 225–26
depression: challenging condition of, 3; PPD (postpartum depression), 27, 228–29; silent epidemic of chronic, 323; as symptom of hormonal imbalance, 43, 46
DHEA (dehydroepiandrosterone), 101, 245
diabetes, 73, 90, 94
diaphragm, 86–87
diarrhea, 108, 175
diet: fiber in, 109–10, 111; FLO Blocker of poor modern, 36–38; gene expression affected by, 40; managing excess sugar in your, 182–83; organic foods as part of your, 36–37; for turning fat-soluble toxins into water-solubles, 114–15; WomanCode Four Days Reset, 114–40; WomanCode Organic Food Essentials, 37. *See also* foods; lifestyle; nutrition
Diet Coke, 100
digestive enzyme, 97
dill seeds, 115
dinners: Four Day Reset, 127, 130, 133, 137; for syncing your cycle, 162, 163
diseases: Alzheimer's, 73; cancer, 73, 85; diabetes, 73, 90; heart disease, 73, 93–94; lymphatic congestion and inflammation-related conditions, 113; STDs (sexually transmitted diseases), 85, 86, 87, 209, 224, 225
Dong quai, 154
dopamine, 238
Duke University, 21, 40
dynamic equation: checking the cues sent by your endocrine system, 171–72; cross-training as part of the, 143–70, 171–73; Heidi Braun's successful use of the, 201; learning how to maximize your hormonal health by using the, 172–73. *See also* endocrine system clues; WomanCode
dynamic equation management: One-on-One with Alisa, 198–200; staying sensitive to your endocrine system clues for, 194–97; Your Daily WomanCode Survival Kit for, 181–85; Your Yearly WomanCode Survival Kit for, 186–94
dysmenorrhea, 3

Easy Beans, 123
egg freezing, 214–15

eggs, 217
elimination system: Alisa's medicine cabinet to improve your, 293; constipation symptom of problem with, 108, 110–11, 139, 175, 296, 298; elevated estrogen levels due to congested, 80; Four Day Reset of WomanCode to improve, 114–40; four pathways of elimination in, 108–13; symptoms of problems with, 43, 59, 175; the WomanCode Zone 4, 67–68, 107–13
endocrine disruptors: beauty products containing, 38–39, 41; excess sugar, 172, 182–83; late-night carb overload, 184–85; skipped meals, 172, 181–82; too much alcohol, 173, 183–84; toxic cleaning products, 134–35, 225. *See also* FLO Blockers
endocrine system: "chemical language" used by your, 45, 48; circadian rhythms of the, 101, 104; cracking the WomanCode for a healthy, 61–63; description and functions of the, 44; dynamic equation of checking in with cues sent by, 171–72; Four Day Reset of WomanCode to recalibrate your, 114–40; functional standpoint on, 145; "lady parts" of the, 60; learning to understand your, 44–46, 55–61; major glands, organs, and hormones of the, 62–63; nourishing your post-pregnancy, 227; WomanCode method to balance the, 3–6; WomanCode Zones on the, 63–69. *See also* GI system; hormones
endocrine system clues: adrenal-related, 53, 174–75; Alisa's medicine cabinet to treat specific, 292–94; blood sugar-related, 59, 78–83, 98–99, 174; elimination-related, 43, 59, 175; FLO Blocker of misinformation about, 33–34, 53–54; learning to tap into the WomanCode signals provided by, 41–42, 69–70, 71, 73; medicinal foods to treat specific, 297–99; metabolism and stress-related, 43; overview of symptoms that act as, 41–43, 53–55; reproductive organs-related, 43, 175–76; staying sensitive vs. desensitized to your, 54, 194–97; WomanCode-approved products to treat specific, 295–96. *See also* dynamic equation; hormonal imbalance; *specific reproduction-related symptoms*
endometriosis, 1, 32, 35, 176
energy. *See* libido
Environmental Protection Agency (EPA), 49
epigenetics, 40

epinephrine (adrenaline), 102–3
estrogen: DHEA precursor to, 101; health
    benefits of sex for, 245; hormonal
    balance of, 45; hypothalamus scan
    for, 69; menstrual cycle governed by,
    144, 148, 152, 154; mismanaged blood
    sugar and elevated levels of, 78–80;
    supplements to increase, 219; syncing
    sex drive with cycle and levels of, 242,
    243. See also hormones
estrogen-dependent diseases, 35
estrogen metabolism, 156
"every meal, every day" concept: blood
    sugar management using, 89; for
    selecting the foods you eat, 65
excess sugar in diet, 182–83
exercise: adrenal fatigue and, 102–3; during
    four phases of menstrual cycle, 147, 149,
    151–52, 154, 163–64; Pilates, 152, 164;
    self-assessing your masculine/feminine
    balance in, 265; strength-training, 102,
    103; yoga, 62, 102, 103, 147, 164, 184,
    255; Your Daily WomanCode Survival Kit
    tips for managing, 181, 183, 184, 185
external stressors, 106

fallopian tubes, 60
family-time events, 191–94
fast burners, 92–93
fat cells: fat-soluble toxins storage in,
    114–15; mismanaged blood sugar as
    cause of, 78–79
fatigue: blood sugar mismanagement cause
    of, 81–83, 98–99; low libido as cause
    of, 27, 81–83; managing blood sugar all
    day to avoid, 96–98; medicinal foods to
    reduce, 298; WomanCode-approved
    products for, 296
fat-soluble toxins, 109–10, 114–15
female condom, 85, 86
feminine energy: characteristics of, 260;
    comparing masculine and, 258–59;
    Daphne Blake's success in revitalizing
    her, 280; engaging your, 59, 267–82;
    five-point star for FLO Living and your,
    275–79, 281; K.C. Baker's success in
    revitalizing her, 282; One-on-One with
    Alisa on, 281; principles of, 269–72,
    285; rebirthing through WomanCode's
    revitalization of, 272–75; self-assessment
    of masculine/feminine balance, 263–67;
    signs of excess masculine energy in
    women, 260–63; sourcing your, 289;
    WomanCode protocol for healing
    through, 267–68. See also libido;
    women

feminine energy principles: on being my
    own authority, 271–72; on conscious and
    collaborative relationships, 270–71; on
    leadership, 270; on living in harmony
    with my biochemistry and self-care,
    269; on pleasure, 270; on receiving, 271;
    360-degree emotional expression, 269
fertility: CAM therapies to improve, 26–30;
    Kathryn Hiller's success in restoring her,
    72
fertility optimization: cultivating a creative
    and fertile mind-set for, 219–22; fertility-
    boosting foods and supplements,
    213–15; health coaching in first steps
    for, 210–13; Katie Reimer's success
    with, 223; Lisa Marie Rice's success in,
    228–29; nourishing your post-pregnancy
    endocrine system for continued, 227;
    One-on-One with Alisa on, 229–30;
    top four recommendations for, 225–26,
    228; WomanCode protocol for, 26–27,
    206–10. See also infertility
fiber, 109–10, 111
Fiber Smart, 139
fibrocystic breasts, 32, 43, 46
fibroids: challenging condition of, 3; silent
    epidemic of, 1, 31, 32, 176; as symptom
    of hormonal imbalance, 43
fight-or-flight response, 66, 101–3
fish and salmon recipes, 124
FLO Blockers: cultural conditioning, 34–35;
    disrupting our endocrine system, 55;
    identifying your own biggest, 50;
    misinformation about your hormones,
    33–34, 53–54; noting the health effects
    of succumbing to, 176–77; our modern
    diet and desire for quick-fix healing
    solutions, 36–38; our toxic environment
    and lifestyle, 35. See also endocrine
    disrupters
FLO Living, as changing the paradigm of
    women's healthcare, 3–6
FLOliving.com: dramatic results of clients
    through support of, 210, 261–63, 284;
    free reset support extras available
    at, 140; online resources available at,
    285–86; origins and mission of, 3, 23,
    274, 284; sharing your story through, 287
FLO Living: description of, 42; five-point
    star for, 275–79, 281; how menstruation,
    fertility, and libido impact, 33; how the
    WomanCode enables you to participate
    in, 10–11; join us on Facebook, 128,
    131; join us on twitter, 288; learning
    to stay in the, 283–87; recreating the
    personal one-on-one sessions at the,

25; sharing the, 287–88; sourcing your power through, 289; women engaged in, 46–47. *See also* health coaching

FLO Living Center: feminine energy as part of the, 261–63; knowledge gained from working with patients of the, 3, 6, 10. *See also* Success Stories

FLO Living online community, 286

flossing/dental health, 225–26

Focus on Digestion, 127, 130, 133, 137. *See also* GI system

follicular phase of menstrual cycle: Foods for Your Cycle during, 159–60, 209–10; overview of the, 146–47; sample meal plans during, 161; syncing your sex drive with, 242

Food Energetics (Gangé), 155

foods: alcohol consumption, 43, 183–84, 189–91, 298; blue/black and yellow/orange, 249; "every meal, every day" concept for selecting, 65; fertility-boosting supplements and, 213–19; Foods for Your Cycle, 146–47, 149, 151, 153–54, 155–56, 157, 159–63, 209–10; issues with dairy and wheat, 196–99; nurturing the adrenal glands, 249; organic, 36–37; soy products, 160–61, 299; supporting hormone balance with medicinal, 297–99; top-ten favorite fertility-boosting, 217–18; WomanCode Four Days Reset, 114–40; WomanCode Organic Food Essentials on, 37; Your Daily WomanCode Survival Kit tips for managing, 181, 182–83, 185. *See also* carbs; diet; meal plans; recipes; supplements

Four Days Reset. *See* WomanCode Four Days Reset

fruits: Foods for Your Cycle, 159, 210; as medicinal foods to treat hormonal symptoms, 298; for turning fat-soluble toxins into water-solubles, 115; WomanCode Organic Food Essentials on, 37

Fruit Salad (only for breakfast), 120

FSH (follicle-stimulating hormone), 63, 69, 144, 146, 218, 242, 319

fun. *See* pleasure

functional medicine, 17

functional nutrition, 19–20

fuzzy-headedness, 27

Gagné, Steve, 155

genetic factors: body reaction to estrogen determined by, 79–80; how our life is impacted by, 40–41

Getting to Thriving, 127, 130, 134, 138

GI system: irritable bowel syndrome (IBS), 3, 43, 46, 108, 175; problems with your, 108. *See also* endocrine system; Focus on Digestion

Glucophage, 16

glucose: how carbs (refined carbohydrates) breaks down into, 64–65, 88–89; how fast versus slow burners process, 79, 92–93; hypoglycemia triggered by low, 90–92, 96, 105; tips for all-day management of blood sugar and, 96–98. *See also* blood sugar

glucose intolerance, 40

gluten sensitivity, 196–97, 199

glycogen, 65

grains: Foods for Your Cycle, 159; Four Day Reset recipes, 122; as medicinal food, 298, 299

Green Drink, 125

greens/salad: as fertility-boosting food, 217; as medicinal foods to treat hormonal symptoms, 297–98; recipes for, 120–21

Groningen University (the Netherlands), 40

grooming products, 38–39

growth hormones, 45

gym locker metaphor, 77–78

Harvard Business Review, 220–21

Hauschka-trained professionals, 18

headaches, 41, 43, 195, 245

health: establishing short-term and long-term goals for, 177; as one of the star dimensions, 276, 277; post-pregnancy, 27, 227–29; sexual, 85, 209, 224–28, 253; Top-Ten Health Benefits of Sex for women, 245; as the ultimate experiment, 176–79

health coaching: for first steps in fertility optimization, 210–13; gradual acceptance into mainstream medicine, 21–22; origins and early history of, 21. *See also* FLO Living; Success Stories

heart disease, 73, 93–94

herbalism, 30

high blood pressure, 16, 94, 113

high blood sugar signs, 174

Hiller, Kathryn, 72

holidays, 191–94

honey, 217

hormonal imbalance: birth control pills used to treat, 14, 16, 81, 82–85; decoding the clues to your, 42–43, 71, 73; "fixing" versus healing, 23; how the body compensates for, 45–46; medicinal foods for symptoms of, 297–99; using

hormonal imbalance, *continued*
  sex to heal your, 244–47; symptoms of,
  41–43, 53–55; WomanCode method
  addressing underlying reasons for, 3.
  See also endocrine system clues
hormonal imbalance causes: congestion
  throughout the pathways of elimination,
  59; lifestyle that works against your
  menstrual cycle, 59; mismanaged
  blood sugar, 59; overexertion of the
  adrenal glands, 59; separation from your
  feminine energy, 59
Hormonal Sync System (online tool), 285,
  288
hormone balance: how the body
  compensates to maintain, 45–46;
  learning about the WomanCode
  protocol for, 2–6, 24–25; what
  chronobiology teaches us about,
  20; what is required for, 45. *See also*
  WomanCode
hormone replacement therapy, 1, 16. *See
  also* the Pill
hormones: ACTH (adrenocorticotropic
  hormone), 65–66, 100;
  adrenocorticotropic hormone
  (ACTH), 63; aldosterone, 101;
  cortisol, 99, 101, 103, 239–40; DHEA
  (dehydroepiandrosterone), 101, 245;
  epinephrine (adrenaline), 102–3; follicle-
  stimulating hormone (FSH), 63, 69, 144,
  146, 148, 218, 242, 319; during four
  phases of menstrual cycle, 146, 148,
  150, 152; governing menstrual cycle,
  144; learning the "five-step system" to
  rebalance your, 2–6; luteinizing hormone
  (LH), 63, 69, 144, 148, 218, 219, 242;
  misinformation about, 33–34; oxytocin,
  239; parathyroid hormone (PTH), 63, 67;
  progesterone, 69, 144, 150, 152, 154;
  sexual responses and role of, 237–41,
  242–43, 244; testosterone, 45, 101,
  144, 150, 242, 243; thyroid-stimulating
  hormone (TSH), 63; wide-spread physical
  impact of, 1–2. *See also* endocrine
  system; estrogen
"Hot Mama Hormones" (lecture), 231–32
house-cleaning products, 134–35, 225
HPA (hypothalamic-pituitary-adrenal) axis,
  35, 65–66, 100, 212, 219
HPO (hypothalamic-pituitary-ovarian) axis,
  69
HPV (human papillomavirus), 1
hunger hormones, 45
hydration, 116
hyperglycemia, 96

hyperthyroidism, 27, 32
hypoglycemia (low blood sugar), 90–92, 96,
  105, 174, 296
hypothalamus: endocrine system role of the,
  62–63; health benefits of sex for, 245;
  HPA (hypothalamic-pituitary-adrenal)
  axis, 35, 65–66, 100, 212, 219; HPO
  (hypothalamic-pituitary-ovarian) axis,
  69; as "lady part," 60; during menstrual
  cycle, 146; relationship of elimination
  system to functioning of, 68; stress and
  response by, 65–66
hypothyroidism, 27, 43
hysterectomies, 1, 32

Immune Booster, 125
immune-strengthening products, 294
infertility: blood sugar mismanagement
  and, 80–81; challenging condition of, 3;
  Clomid to treat, 16, 223; egg freezing
  in case of, 214–15; high rates of, 1;
  how WomanCode can identify hidden
  causes of, 208–9; IVF treatment for, 16,
  27, 206, 207, 214–15, 218, 228; silent
  epidemic of, 32, 205–6; STDs (sexually
  transmitted diseases) causing, 224,
  225; understanding chemical, radiation,
  and bacterial factors in, 224–26, 228;
  unexplained, 43, 46. *See also* fertility
  optimization; reproductive organs
information vacation, 271–72
insomnia: as symptom of hormonal
  imbalance, 41, 43, 46; WomanCode
  protocol solution to, 27
Institute for Integrative Nutrition, 21
insulin resistance, 40
internal stressors: description of, 105; Four
  Day Reset of WomanCode to reduce,
  114–40
in-vitro fertilization (IVF), 16, 27, 206, 207,
  214–15, 218, 228
irritability, 96, 298
irritable bowel syndrome (IBS), 3, 43, 46,
  108, 175
IUDs, 87

journaling: during Four Day Reset, 127, 130,
  134, 138; during menstrual phase, 153
Journal of Clinical Investigation, 91
Journal of Sexual Medicine, 254
*Journal of the American College of
  Cardiology*, 94
The Joy of Sex (Comfort), 12

Kent, Naomi, 95
kidneys, 60

"lady parts," 60

large intestine: elimination pathway through the liver and, 108–11; as "lady part," 60; symptoms of problems with, 175; WomanCode Zone 4: skin, lymphatic system, liver and, 67–68

leadership principle of feminine energy, 270

leafy greens, 120–21, 217, 297–98

legumes/beans, 159, 298, 299

LH (luteinizing hormone), 63, 69, 144, 148, 218, 219, 242

libido: blood sugar mismanagement causing low, 81–83, 98–99; CAM therapies to improve, 26–30; defined as ability to give and receive pleasure, 251–53; Fran Mooney's success in improving her, 241; how the Pill can lower your, 254; One-on-One with Alisa on your, 254–55; separation from your feminine energy and, 59; symptoms related to low, 43, 178; WomanCode protocol to improve your sex drive and, 27, 231–35. *See also* adrenal fatigue; feminine energy

lifestyle: endocrine disruptors in beauty products, 38–39; during four phases of menstrual cycle, 146, 148–49, 150–51, 152–53; hormonal imbalance due to toxic, 45; increasing your personal creativity as part of your, 219–22, 278; as one of the star dimensions, 276, 277; toxic environment and, 35, 45; working against your menstrual cycle, 59; Your Daily WomanCode Survival Kit on your, 182, 183, 184, 185; Your Yearly WomanCode Survival Kit on your, 186–94. *See also* diet

Lively Lentils, 123

liver: elimination pathway through the large intestine and, 108–11; fat-soluble toxins removed by, 109–10, 114–15; as one of the "lady parts," 60; symptoms of problems with, 175; WomanCode Zone 1: blood sugar group–pancreas and, 64–65, 79–98; WomanCode Zone 4: lymphatic system, skin, large intestine and, 67–68

liver cleansing medleys recipes, 120–21

low blood sugar (hypoglycemia), 90–92, 96, 105, 174, 296

low libido: challenging condition of, 3; Daphne Blake's success in improving her, 280; Fran Mooney's success in improving her, 241; how the Pill effects, 254; medicinal foods to increase, 298; symptoms related to, 27, 43, 178

lunches: Four Day Reset, 126, 129, 132, 137; for syncing your cycle, 162, 163; tips for managing blood sugar during, 96–97

lupus, 113

luteal phase of cycle: Foods for Your Cycle during, 159–60, 209–10; overview of, 150–52; sample meal plans during, 162; syncing your sex drive with, 243

lymphatic system: elimination pathway through the, 112–13; as "lady part," 60; sex benefits to the, 245; symptoms of problems with, 175; WomanCode Zone 4: liver, skin, large intestine and, 67–68

magnesium supplement, 227

Magnificent Mung Beans, 123

makeup toxins, 38

male condom, 85, 86

masculine energy: characteristics of, 259; comparing feminine and, 258–59; self-assessment of masculine/feminine balance, 263–67; women with excess of, 260–63

massage therapy, 29, 221

McKinsey & Company study, 220

meal plans: Four Days Reset activities and, 126–40; online library of suggestions for, 286; self-assessing your masculine/feminine balance in, 265; for syncing your cycle, 162–63. *See also* foods

meats. *See* protein

medicinal food list, 297–99

meditation, 62

menopause, 27

menstrual cycle: Alisa's medicine cabinet to support your, 293; the amazing process of the, 20; CAM therapies to improve difficult, 28–30; cycle syncing during four phases of the, 143–70, 171–73, 241–44; five hormones that govern your, 144; "The Period Club" of friends experiencing first, 12–13; "Seeing Red" on your menstrual flow, 154, 208; symptoms of hormonal issues of, 43; WomanCode protocol for healthy, 26. *See also* reproductive organs

menstrual cycle syncing: Emily Bohannon's success with, 158; exercise and, 147, 149, 151–52, 154, 163–64; Foods for Your Cycle, 146–47, 149, 151, 153–54, 155–56, 157, 159–63, 209–10; during the four cycle phases, 145–54, 162–63; issues to consider for, 143–45; One-on-One with Alisa on, 170; practicality of planning your life around, 166; rebuilding your relationship with your body through,

menstrual cycle syncing, *continued*
167–70, 171–73; stepping-stones for,
165, 167; when you're on the Pill, 168–69;
why it works, 157; of your sex drive and,
241–44
menstrual phase: Foods for Your Cycle
during, 154–55, 159–60, 209–10;
interpreting flow during the, 154–55;
overview of the, 152–53; sample meal
plan during, 163; syncing your sex drive
with, 243
menstruation problems: the author's
personal experience with, 13–16; birth
control pill used to treat, 14, 81, 82–85;
CAM therapies to improve, 28–30;
Kathryn Hiller's success in reducing
her, 72; lifestyle that causes, 59;
mismanaged blood sugar linked to,
79–83; PMS, 43, 144, 208, 258, 282;
silent epidemic of, 1, 31; symptoms of,
43, 46, 299; understanding why you
have, 79–80; WomanCode protocol to
help with, 26
metabolic syndrome: signs of, 40; as
symptom of hormonal problems, 43
metabolism: comparing fast versus slow
burners, 79, 92–93; symptoms of
problems with, 43
micronutrients, 156
midafternoon: Four Day Reset snacks for,
129–30, 132–33, 137; tips for managing
blood sugar, 97
migraines, 43, 245
mind-body connection, 62
mind-set: benefits of adopting new, 142–43;
cultivating a creative and fertile, 219–22;
discarding your static, 141–42
miscarriages, 27, 80
monounsatured fats, 213–14, 216
mood swings, 299
Mooney, Fran, 241
morning, tips for managing blood sugar, 96
Mung Bean Minestrone, 119–20

National Academy of Sciences, 177
National Institutes of Health, 31
naturopathy, 29
neurotransmitters, 238
nitric oxide, 239, 245
Northrup, Christiane, 257, 258
nurture your adrenals: foods that, 249;
WomanCode Protocol, 59, 98–113.
See also adrenal fatigue
nutrition: functional, 19–20; micronutrients,
156. *See also* diet; supplements
nuts, 159

obesity: metabolic syndrome and, 40,
43; mismanaged blood sugar as one
cause of, 78–79, 98–99. *See also* weight
problems
omega-3 fatty acids, 209, 213, 216, 218
omega-3 oil, 155, 227, 294
One-on-One with Alisa: on dynamic
equation, 198–200; on feminine energy,
281; on fertility optimization, 229–30;
how to use these, 25; on identifying your
biggest FLO Blocker, 50; on improving
your libido, 254–55; questions to ask
on endocrine system and WomanCode
Zones, 73; on reducing stress, 106–7;
on stabilizing your blood sugar, 98; on
syncing your cycle, 170
organic food, 36–37
orgasms: body during, 235–36; low libido
impact on, 27, 178; stress of lack of
regular, 105
orthorexia (eating disorder), 36–37
ovaries: airport security scanning potentially
damaging, 226; Heidi Braun's success in
healing her, 201; hormone-sensitivity of,
68; HPO (hypothalamic-pituitary-ovarian)
axis, 69; as "lady part," 60; luteal phase
of cycle and the, 150–52; pre-conception
feeding of nutrient-dense foods to your,
215
The Ovary Oath, 49
ovulation, 80
ovulatory phase of cycle: Foods for Your
Cycle during, 159–60, 209–10; overview
of the, 148–49; sample meal plans
during, 162; syncing your sex drive with,
242–43
oxytocin, 239
Oz, Mehmet, 21

painful/difficult/heavy periods. *See*
menstruation problems
pancreas: as one of the "lady parts," 60;
WomanCode Zone 1: blood sugar
group–liver and, 64–65, 79–98
The Parable of the Leaping Cricket, 138
parathyroid: PTH (parathyroid hormone)
produced by, 63, 67; WomanCode
Zone 3: metabolic group–thyroid and,
66–67
PCOS (polycycstic ovary syndrome):
author's diagnosis with, 15–17, 54;
author's journey to treating her own,
17–20; challenging condition of, 3;
Emily Whyte's success story on, 51–52;
genetic predisposition to, 40–41; Lisa
Marie Rice's success story on, 228–29;

mismanaged blood sugar contributing to, 79–80; ovulation prevented by, 80; sharing the author's protocol to other women, 21–23; silent epidemic of, 1, 31; as symptom of hormonal imbalance, 43. See also reproductive organs; Stein-Leventhal disease

pelvic pain/cramping, 299

perimenopause, 27, 80, 207, 220–21

phtahalates (DPB, DEHP), 35, 38

physical inactivity/muscle tightness, 105

PID (pelvic inflammatory disease), 224

Pilates, 152, 164

the Pill: cycle-syncing if you're on the, 168–69; menstrual problems treated with, 14, 81; as no protection against STDs, 224; PCOS treated by HRT in the form of, 16; the truth about taking, 82–85; your libido and, 254. See also hormone replacement therapy

pituitary gland: HPA (hypothalamic-pituitary-adrenal) axis, 35, 65–66, 100, 212, 219; HPO (hypothalamic-pituitary-ovarian) axis, 69; as "lady part," 60; TSH (thyroid-stimulating hormone) sent out by, 63

pleasure: creating a recipe to increase your, 248–49; feminine energy principle on, 270; learning to give and receive, 251–53; as one of the star dimensions, 276, 279; turning yourself on, 247–50

PMS symptoms, 43, 144, 208, 258, 282

polychlorinated biphenyl (PCB), 35

postmenopausal sex life, 246

post-pregnancy health: postpartum depression (PPD), 27, 228–29; recommendations for, 227

prefrontal cortex, 91, 177–78

pregnancy: health after, 27, 227–29; how WomanCode can help maintain your, 208; during perimenopause, 220–21; progesterone to maintain, 80

Principles of Feminine Energy, 269–72, 285

progesterone: hypothalamus scan for, 69; menstrual cycle governed by, 144, 150, 152, 154; supplements to increase, 219; syncing sex drive with cycle and levels of, 242, 243

protein: Foods for Your Cycle, 159, 210; medicinal foods for hormonal symptoms, 298, 299; recipes for daily, 123; WomanCode Organic Food Essentials on, 37

quick-fix solutions, 36–38

Quick Veggie Soup, 119

Quinoa Recipe, 122

Rainbow Light's Advanced Enzyme System, 97

Raw Kale Salad, 121

receiving: developing capacity for giving and, 251–53; feminine energy principle of, 271

recipes, See also foods

Reimer, Katie, 223

relationships: conscious and collaborative, 270–71; improving your sexual responses regardless of, 234–35; learning to give and receive in your, 251–53; self-assessing your masculine/feminine balance in, 265; social connection and community, 276, 278

reproductive organs: ovaries, 60, 68–69, 150–52; signs of imbalance in, 175; symptoms of problems with, 176. See also infertility; menstrual cycle; PCOS (polycycstic ovary syndrome)

rheumatoid arthritis, 113

Rice, Lisa Marie, 228–29

rice/grains recipes, 122

right to choose principle, 271–72

safe sex practices, 85, 224, 225

salad/greens recipes, 120–21

Sautéed Escarole, 121

seafood: fertility-boosting, 218; fish and salmon recipes, 124; Foods for Your Cycle, 160, 210

self-care, 269, 276, 277

sensitivity (increasing capacity for), 194–97

serotonin, 238

sex: ability to give and receive pleasure during, 251–53; healing your hormones through, 244, 246–47; during postmenopausal years, 246; The Ten WomanCode Keys to Healthy Sexual Self-Expression during, 253; top-ten health benefits for women, 245

sex drive: cycle-sync your, 241–44; feedback loop of your, 233–34; Fran Mooney's success in improving her, 241; One-on-One with Alisa on improving your, 254–55; WomanCode protocol to improve, 27, 231–35

sexual health: confirming your, 209; optimizing fertility by improving your, 224–28; safe sex practices for, 85, 224, 225; The Ten WomanCode Keys to Healthy Sexual Self-Expression and, 253; top four recommendations for improving, 225–26, 228

sexual responses: creating your own pleasure recipe to improve, 248–49;

sexual responses, *continued*
four stages of, 235–37; learning to
turn yourself on, 247–50; One-on-One
with Alisa on improving your, 254–55;
orgasms, 27, 105, 178, 235–36; role of
your brain in, 237–41
skin: acne/rosacea/eczema conditions of the,
1, 3, 43, 53, 99, 108, 175, 282, 295, 297;
bathing in Epsom salts and essential oils,
139–40; elimination pathway through
the, 111–12; symptoms of problems with,
175; WomanCode-approved products
for the, 295; WomanCode Zone 4: liver
and large intestine, lymphatic system,
and, 67–68
skipped meals, 172, 181–82
sleep patterns: body fat related to, 40;
insomnia, 27, 41, 43, 46; stress of
irregular, 105
slow burners, 79, 92–93
small intestines, 60
snacks: Four Day Reset early morning,
126, 129, 132, 136–37; Four Day Reset
midafternoon, 129–30, 132–33, 137
social connection and community, 276, 278
sodium lauryl ether sulfate (SLES), 38
sodium lauryl sulfate (SLS), 38
soup recipes, 119–20
soy products, 160–61, 299
Spring Mix Salad, 120
Spring Style Pilaf, 122
SSRIs (selective serotonin reuptake
inhibitors), 238
star: five points of the, 275–76; how to use
the, 277–79; unleashing your organic
feminine power to become a, 279, 281
STDs (sexually transmitted diseases), 85, 86,
87, 209, 224, 225
Steam Sautéed Veggies, 121
Stein-Leventhal disease, 15. *See also* PCOS
(polycystic ovarian syndrome)
strength-training, 102, 103
stress: adrenal fatigue and effects of, 99–
100; and blood sugar mismanagement
causing fatigue, 81–83, 98–99; body
checks and balances for hormonal
imbalance due to, 45; circadian rhythmic
disruption due to, 104; fight-or-flight
response to, 66, 101–3; Four Day Reset
of WomanCode to reduce internal,
114–40; HPA (hypothalamic-pituitary-
adrenal) axis response to, 35, 65–66,
100, 212, 219; internal and external
stressors, 105–6; the natural way to
sooth, 104–6; One-on-One with Alisa on

reducing, 106–7; symptoms of problems
with, 43. *See also* adrenal glands
Success Stories: Daphne Blake, 280; Emily
Bohannon, 158; Emily Whyte, 51–52;
Fran Mooney, 241; Heidi Braun, 201;
K.C. Baker, 282; Kathryn Hiller, 72; Katie
Reimer, 223; Lisa Marie Rice, 228–29;
Naomi Kent, 95; sharing your own, 287.
See also FLO Living Center; health
coaching
sunflower seeds, 217
supplements: Alisa's medicine cabinet
recommendations for, 291–94; hormone-
enhancing, 218–19; for improving your
sex drive, 248; menstrual cycle and
helpful, 154, 155; post-pregnancy, 227.
See also Alisa's medicine cabinet; foods;
nutrition
support, resources, and abundance, 276,
277–78
symptoms. *See* endocrine system clues
syncing your cycle. *See* menstrual cycle
syncing

tender breasts, 46
The Ten WomanCode Keys to Healthy
Sexual Self-Expression, 253
testosterone: DHEA precursor to, 101;
hormonal balance of, 45; menstrual cycle
governed by, 144, 148, 150; syncing sex
drive with cycle and levels of, 242, 243
thyroid: as "lady part," 60; WomanCode
Zone 3: metabolic group–parathyroid
and, 66–67
thyroid issues: challenging condition of, 3;
silent epidemic of, 1, 32; symptoms of,
53; WomanCode protocol to improve,
27; X-ray damage to thyroid, 226
thyroid-stimulating hormone (TSH), 63
The Today sponge, 86
Top-Ten Health Benefits of Sex, 245
toxic environment/lifestyle: as FLO Blocker,
35; hormonal imbalance due to, 45;
house-cleaning products, 134–35
Toxic Substances Control Act (1976), 49
Traditional Chinese Medicine (TCM): blue/
black foods and yellow/orange foods of,
249; as framework for understanding the
body, 19; on observations of the health
of our own bodies, 107; turmeric used
in, 218
trampoline (rebounder), 113
transvaginal ultrasound, 15
turmeric, 218, 294
twitter FLO Living account, 288

unexplained infertility, 43, 46
urinary tract infections (UTI), 95, 209, 296, 299
uterus, 60

vacations: taking an information, 271–72; taking a WomanCode, 186–87
vaginal contraceptive film, 87
vegetables: Foods for Your Cycle, 159, 210; greens/salad recipes, 120–21; as medicinal foods to treat hormonal symptoms, 297–99; for turning fat-soluble toxins into water-solubles, 115; WomanCode Organic Food Essentials on, 37; yellow/orange foods, 249
vitamin B-complex, 155, 184, 227, 293
vitamin C, 184, 248
vitamin D3, 209, 227
vulva, 60

walking/jogging exercise, 102
water consumption, 116, 297, 298, 299
weight problems: challenging condition of, 1, 3; fat cells holding onto fat-soluble toxins causing, 114–15; mismanaged blood sugar as one cause of, 78–79, 98–99; post-pregnancy, 27; as symptom of hormonal imbalance, 43, 46. See also obesity
Weil, Andrew, 21
What to Expect When You're Expecting (Sandee et al.), 12
Whyte, Emily, 51–52
willpower, 90–91
WomanCode: becoming an ambassador for, 286–87; common-sense basis of, 47; description of, 42, 48; fertility preservation and enhancement through the, 26–27; four days to reset your, 114–40; gym locker metaphor of, 77–78; healing your endocrine system through, 56–61; how FLO Living is enabled by the, 10–11; introduction to the, 3–6, 10; "lady parts" according to the, 60; learning to crack the, 61–63; libido restoration and improvement through the, 27; period perfection through the, 26; promise to you about the, 71, 73; rebirthing yourself through the, 272–75; reshaping your personal story through the, 25–26; sharing the FLO and, 287–88, 289; staying in the FLO by living the, 283–87;

tapping into the signals of your, 69–70. See also dynamic equation; hormone balance
WomanCode-Approved Products, 38, 295–96
WomanCode five-step protocol: cross-train your menstrual cycle, 59, 143–70, 171–73, 241–44, 293; cumulative process of the, 24–25; engage your feminine energy, 59, 267–82, 289; nurture your adrenals, 59, 98–113, 249, 292; online video session taking your through the, 285; stabilize your blood sugar, 59, 86–98, 114–40, 292; support organs of elimination, 59, 107–13, 114–40, 293
WomanCode Organic Food Essentials, 37
WomanCode Reset: Day 1: meal plan and activities, 126–28; Day 2: meal plan and activities, 129–31; Day 3: meal plan and activities, 132–35; Day 4: meal plan and activities, 136–40; FLOliving.com information on, 140; food and mind prep for, 117–19; introduction to the, 114–16; recipes for, 119–25; shopping list for the, 116–17; staying hydrated during the, 116
WomanCode Survival Kit: daily, 181–86; yearly, 186–94. See also endocrine disruptors
WomanCode Zones: 1: blood sugar group—pancreas and liver, 64–65, 79–98; 2: stress group—HPA axis, 65–66, 98–113; 3: metabolic group—thyroid and parathyroid, 66–67; 4: elimination group—liver and large intestine, lymphatic system, and skin, 67–68, 107–13; 5: reproductive group—hypothalamic-pituitary-ovarian (HPO) axis, 69
women: cultural condition of, 34–35; misinformed about their own hormones, 33–34; signs of excess masculine energy in, 260–63; Top-Ten Health Benefits of Sex for, 245. See also feminine energy
Women's Bodies, Women's Wisdom (Northrup), 257
work demands, 187–89

xenoestrogens, 35

Yearly WomanCode Survival Kit, 186–94
yeast infections, 46, 296, 299
yellow/orange foods, 249
yoga, 62, 102, 103, 147, 164, 184, 255

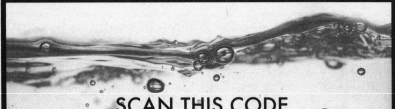

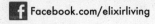